MAYO CLINIC

—ON—

DIGESTIVE HEALTH

Stephen Crane Hauser, M.D.

Medical Editor

Mayo Clinic

Rochester, Minnesota

Mayo Clinic on Digestive Health provides reliable, practical, easy-to-understand information on identifying and managing digestive signs and symptoms and conditions. Much of this information comes directly from the experience of gastroenterologists, hepatologists and other health care professionals at Mayo Clinic. This book is intended to supplement the advice of your personal physician, whom you should consult regarding individual medical conditions. *Mayo Clinic on Digestive Health* does not endorse any company or product. MAYO, MAYO CLINIC and the Mayo triple-shield logo are marks of Mayo Foundation for Medical Education and Research.

Stock photography from Getty Images. The individuals pictured are models, and the photos are used for illustrative purposes only. There's no correlation between the individuals portrayed and the conditions or subjects being discussed.

The endoscopic images on pages 117, 120, 143, 170 and 233 are courtesy of the American Registry of Pathology and the Armed Forces Institute of Pathology, *Atlas of Gastrointestinal Endoscopy & Endoscopic Biopsies* (2000).

Address inquiries to: Mayo Clinic Health Information, Rights and Permissions, 200 First St. SW, Fifth Floor, Centerplace Building, Rochester, MN 55905.

For bulk sales to employers, member groups and health-related companies, contact Mayo Clinic Health Solutions, 200 First St. SW, Rochester, MN 55905, or send an email to *SpecialSalesMayoBooks@mayo.edu*.

Library of Congress Control Number: 2010938898

Printed in the United States of America

Third Edition

1 2 3 4 5 6 7 8 9 10

About digestive conditions

Digestive problems are among the most common reasons people see their doctors. They're also a leading reason why people take medication. For example, next time you visit a pharmacy or grocery store, take note of the array of antacids and acid blockers on display for heartburn. Other common digestive complaints include indigestion, abdominal pain, nausea, diarrhea, constipation and gas.

You may have come to accept these signs and symptoms as natural byproducts of digestion. Often, though, they're your body's way of telling you that something is wrong. The good news is that with early diagnosis, most digestive problems often can be successfully treated or managed.

Within these pages you'll find solid, practical advice to help identify digestive problems before they become more serious. You'll also learn about simple changes you can make to your lifestyle that may reduce the risk of digestive disease. This book is based on the expertise of Mayo Clinic doctors and the advice they give day in and day out in caring for their patients.

About Mayo Clinic

Mayo Clinic is the first and largest integrated, not-for-profit group practice in the world. Doctors from every medical specialty work together to care for patients, joined by common systems and a philosophy that the needs of the patient come first. Over 3,600 physicians and scientists and 50,000 allied staff work at Mayo, which has sites in Rochester, Minn.; Jacksonville, Fla.; and Scottsdale/Phoenix, Ariz. Collectively, Mayo Clinic treats more than 500,000 patients a year.

For more than 100 years, millions of people from all walks of life have found answers at Mayo Clinic. Mayo Clinic works with many insurance companies, does not require a physician referral in most cases and is an in-network provider for millions of people.

With its depth of medical knowledge, experience and expertise, Mayo Clinic occupies an unparalleled position as an award-winning health information resource.

Editorial staff

Medical Editor

Stephen Crane Hauser, M.D.

Director, Health Information

Jay Maxwell

**Senior Product Manager,
Books and Newsletters**

Christopher Frye

Managing Editor

Kevin Kaufman

Editorial Research Librarians

Anthony Cook

Amanda Golden

Deirdre Herman

Proofreading

Miranda Attlesey

Donna Hanson

Creative Director

Wes Weleczki

Art Director

Rick Resnick

Illustration

Michael King

Indexing

Steve Rath

Administrative Assistant

Beverly Steele

Terri Zanto Strausbauch

Contributing editors and reviewers

Suresh Chari, M.D.

Dawn Francis, M.D.

G. Richard Locke III, M.D.

Joseph Murray, M.D.

Jennifer K. Nelson, R.D.

William Sanchez, M.D.

Jacalyn See, R.D.

William Tremaine, M.D.

Cover design by Daryl Luepke

Preface

Your digestive system may seem easy to understand. You put food in your mouth, and digestion breaks it down in your stomach so that all the nutritious parts are absorbed and waste is eliminated. Sounds simple, doesn't it?

In fact, your digestive system is incredibly complex — part transportation system and part processing plant that requires the efficient function of many different organs to transform everything you eat and drink into a form that fuels your good health. It's easy to imagine the problems that might occur.

An obvious point that can be made about *Mayo Clinic on Digestive Health* is that there's information in this book that will be important to you. It's likely that you've experienced temporary discomfort from heartburn, diarrhea, constipation, nausea or excess gas. Everyone does at some point in life.

It's also possible that you're dealing with a common digestive condition, such as gastroesophageal reflux disease, peptic ulcers or gallstones. You may be looking for help in managing a long-term condition, such as lactose intolerance or Crohn's disease. This book addresses a wide range of digestive topics, provid-

ing a context for what it takes to keep your system healthy and what happens when something goes wrong.

Mayo Clinic on Digestive Health describes signs and symptoms, causes, diagnostic procedures, and treatment options for the most common digestive conditions, as well as preventive actions to consider. Too often, people wait too long before seeking help from their doctors. In general, the earlier you address a problem, the easier it is to prevent it from becoming serious.

Here's hoping that this book can help you enjoy a higher quality of life with fcwcr digestive concerns. And here's wishing you good digestion!

Stephen Crane Hauser, M.D.

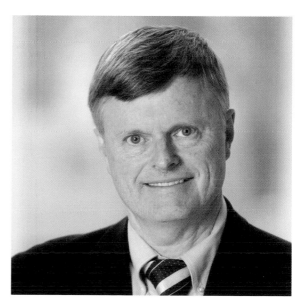

Table of contents

Part 2

Part 1

Digestive health basics

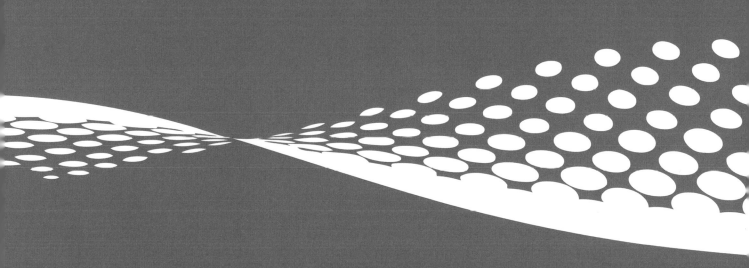

Chapter 1

Your digestive system

Heartburn, cramps, bloating, nausea, diarrhea, constipation — these are just a few of the ways that your digestive system lets you know when things aren't quite right. Try as you might to stick to a daily routine, the anxiety and discomfort caused by these signs and symptoms are hard to ignore. You may look to over-the-counter medications for relief but this measure is rarely a long-term solution.

Generally, the signs and symptoms will diminish after a few hours but for some people, digestive distress persists and becomes a constant concern. The problem may have many possible causes, including infection, inflammation or abnormal blockage in the digestive tract. Regardless, the signs and symptoms don't go away, no matter what you may do to relieve them.

It's estimated that about 1 in 3 Americans — perhaps even more — experiences some form of persistent digestive problem. You can see evidence of how common these problems are with a visit to your local drugstore or grocery. Shelves are lined with an impressive array of medicines and supplements to treat digestive conditions, including antacids, acid blockers, laxatives, fiber supplements and anti-diarrheal agents. Each year Americans spend more than $2 billion to purchase these over-the-counter products.

Although they can often help relieve acute signs and symptoms, over-the-counter medications may not be the complete answer. If you're regularly bothered by periods of indigestion or nausea or cramps, it's important that you see your doctor.

Knowing the root cause of a digestive problem may help reduce anxiety, put you more at ease in social interactions, and allow you and your doctor to work together on a plan to manage the condition and possibly even to cure it. Early action on your part may also prevent a serious digestive condition from becoming life-threatening.

How digestion works

Digestion is one of the critical functions that your body has to perform in order to survive. Food supplies the necessary nutrients that provide your cells with sustenance and energy, allowing your body to grow and develop, and to repair and maintain itself.

Food moves through your body along the digestive tract, a series of hollow, connected organs including the esophagus, stomach, small intestine and colon — together they form a long, convoluted passageway extending from the mouth to the anus, where solid waste exits the body. Organs such as the salivary glands, pancreas, liver and gallbladder also serve essential functions in the digestive process.

When you put food in your mouth, the food must be transformed before it can be used to nourish your body. That's the primary function of digestion — to break food down into smaller components and change it chemically so that nutrients can be extracted and absorbed into your bloodstream (while the remainder is eliminated as waste). The breakdown occurs primarily through the action of digestive juices in your mouth, stomach and intestines, with assistance from the tearing, grinding action of your teeth.

Muscular contractions move food along through successive stages of the digestive process. Valves at critical junctures control the amount of food that can be moved forward and prevent food from moving backward. A network of nerves regulates much of this activity, including the release of enzymes and digestive juices. When food is broken down, nutrients are absorbed into your blood via tiny pores in the intestinal wall. The nutrients are transported in the bloodstream to nourish your body cells.

When things go according to plan, the various organs of your digestive tract perform many specialized functions in an efficient and timely manner. But any complex system comprised of integrated parts carrying multiple respon-

The digestive tract begins at the mouth and ends at the rectum. It includes several vital internal organs.

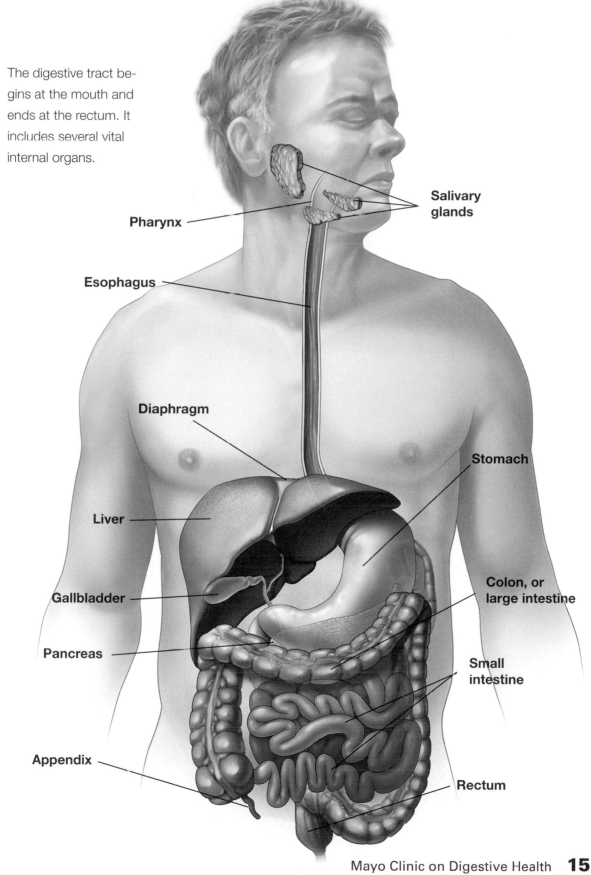

Salivary glands

Pharynx

Esophagus

Diaphragm

Stomach

Liver

Colon, or large intestine

Gallbladder

Pancreas

Small intestine

Appendix

Rectum

sibilities can sometimes break down. Even a slight delay or malfunction may disrupt the entire system. Furthermore, your signs and symptoms may point to any number of possible causes, making a diagnosis difficult (and your life miserable). The tasks at hand for you and your doctor during a medical visit are to identify all the possibilities and — often through a process of elimination — focus on the most likely cause.

The material you've just read is a big picture view of the digestive process. The sections that follow describe the different organs, their functions and relationships to each other. This knowledge may help explain the complexities of the digestive process and why digestive problems are so common.

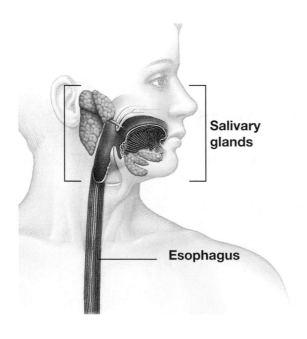

Salivary glands

Esophagus

Salivary glands

Digestion starts even before you take your first bite. The aroma of the food you're about to eat — or even the thought of eating — is enough to get saliva in your mouth flowing. You have three pairs of large salivary glands, in addition to smaller glands in the lining of your mouth.

When you take a bite, your glands pump out saliva containing the enzyme amylase (AM-uh-lase) that begins to chemically break down the food. Your teeth crunch and grind the food, while your tongue mixes it with the saliva. These actions transform a bite of food into a bolus — a soft, moist, rounded mixture suitable for swallowing.

You control many aspects of the digestive process at the beginning — what you put into your mouth, how long you chew it, and when you swallow. But once you swallow, the rest of the digestive process is controlled by your nervous system.

Esophagus

When you swallow, muscles in your mouth and throat propel food through a relaxed ring of muscle (upper esopha-

Appetite, hunger and feeling full

Appetite is that pleasant feeling that lets you know it's time to eat. Hunger comes later, perhaps when you've gone past your normal mealtime and your body tells you so with unpleasant hunger pangs. Appetite and hunger work together to keep you eating regularly.

Your sensations of appetite and hunger are controlled by a part of your brain called the hypothalamus. A portion of the food you eat is converted into blood sugar (glucose). When your blood sugar level drops, the hypothalamus notices and sends nerve impulses along the vagus nerve to your stomach. These impulses trigger the release of gastric juices, and set in motion the muscle contractions that produce hunger pangs. You may hear your stomach rumbling as juices and air pass through your intestines.

If you aren't able to eat right away, these sensations gradually wear off and you may not feel hungry again for several hours. But later in the day, when it's time for your next meal, you may feel famished.

Once you've eaten, your brain recognizes when you're full. As your stomach fills and stretches to its normal capacity, it signals that your hunger has been satisfied.

geal sphincter) that connects the back of your throat (pharynx) to your upper esophagus. The esophagus is a tube, typically about 10 inches long, that connects your throat and stomach.

Gravity alone is not sufficient to move the bolus through the esophagus. Help comes from strong esophageal muscles that move in synchronized waves —

one after another — propelling the food toward your stomach. Muscles behind the swallowed food contract, squeezing it forward, while muscles in front relax to allow the food to advance without resistance. This pattern of progressive contraction and relaxation is called peristalsis (per-ih-STAL-sis) — a muscular action that continues through your entire digestive tract.

As food reaches the lower portion of your esophagus, it approaches the lower esophageal sphincter. When you're not eating, this muscle valve remains tightly closed to keep stomach acid from flowing backward (regurgitating) into your esophagus and causing heartburn. The act of swallowing signals the valve to relax and open in order to let food pass through on its way to your stomach.

Stomach

Your stomach sits in an upper corner of your abdomen, just under your rib cage. A hollow, muscular sac, the typical stomach is about 10 inches long and can expand to hold about a gallon of food and liquid. When your stomach is empty, its tissues fold in on themselves, a bit like a closed accordion. As your stomach fills, the folds disappear.

Your stomach performs two functions in the digestive process. It continues to break food down into smaller pieces, and it acts as a storehouse, gradually releasing food into the small intestine — where most chemical digestion and absorption take place. Generally, it takes your stomach about four hours to empty after a nutritious meal (six hours or more if the meal has a lot of fat).

Even before food arrives, digestive juices in the stomach begin flowing. At the first sight, smell and taste of food, your brain sends messages along the vagus nerve indicating that food will be arriving soon. The messages trigger the release of acetylcholine (as-uh-tul-KO-lene) in your stomach. This chemical sets off a chain reaction that starts your stomach muscles contracting and signals your gastric glands to produce digestive juices.

By the time food arrives from your esophagus, conditions are ready for the next stage of digestion. The muscles in your upper stomach relax to allow a greater volume of food and liquid to enter. The stomach walls, which are lined with three layers of powerful muscles, then begin churning the food, mixing it into smaller and smaller pieces. Gastric juices released from glands lining the walls of your stomach help break down food into a thick, creamy fluid called chyme (kime). In a normal day, your stomach produces 2 to 3 quarts of gastric juices.

Hydrochloric acid is one of many kinds of gastric juice. This acid would be very corrosive in your stomach if it weren't for a layer of sticky mucus clinging to your stomach walls. Hydrochloric acid kills harmful bacteria and microorganisms swallowed with the food. Gastric juices also contain pepsin, a protein-digesting enzyme that works mainly on milk.

Two products that are absorbed directly into your bloodstream from your stomach are aspirin and alcohol, both of which pass quickly through the stomach lining with little trouble.

Once your food is well mixed, rippling waves of muscles in your stomach walls push the stomach contents down toward the pyloric valve, which opens into your small intestine. The pyloric valve, another ring-like sphincter muscle, opens just enough to allow your stomach to release less than an

eighth of an ounce of food at a time into the small intestine. The rest of the contents is held back for more mixing.

Small intestine, pancreas, liver and gallbladder

The small intestine is a winding passage that fills much of your abdomen. It's here that the chemical breakdown of the food you eat is completed, and where most nutrients are absorbed into your bloodstream. The length of the small intestine in most adults is generally about 21 feet long. The small intestine is divided into three parts: duodenum, jejunum and ileum.

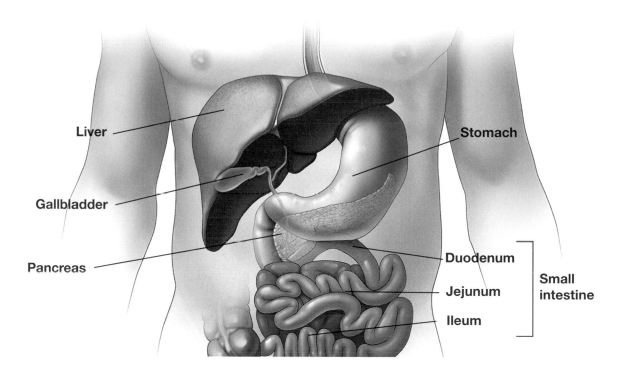

Liver

Gallbladder

Pancreas

Stomach

Duodenum

Jejunum

Ileum

Small intestine

Food released from your stomach passes into the duodenum (doo-o-DEE-num), which is about 12 inches long. The breakdown of food continues in this upper portion of your small intestine. The lining of the duodenum contains enzymes — for example, lactase — that can break down double sugars, such as lactose, into simple sugars, such as glucose and galactose. The digestive juices are channeled into the duodenum from the following organs.

Pancreas

Your pancreas is a soft, pink-colored gland that's located behind the stomach. Shaped a bit like a fish, with a wide head, tapering body and narrow tail, the pancreas is, on average, about 6 inches long and less than 2 inches wide. In addition to making other secretions, the pancreas produces two important types of digestive chemicals. They are:

- The hormones insulin and glucagon, which are secreted into your bloodstream and help regulate your metabolism, including levels of blood sugar (glucose)

- Digestive enzymes that are secreted into your upper duodenum and help break down your main energy sources — proteins, carbohydrates and fats

Liver

Located just under your rib cage on the right side of your abdomen, the liver is a large organ similar in size to a football. The liver is a virtual chemical factory that performs more than 500 functions. Those functions include storing the nutrients from digested food, as well as filtering and processing potentially toxic substances you consume, such as alcohol, chemicals and most medications. The liver also produces bile, a yellowish-green solution that helps break down fat so that it can be absorbed into your blood.

Gallbladder

Your gallbladder is a small, translucent sac that lies adjacent to your liver. The organ is key part of the biliary tract, a system for transporting bile to the small intestine. The gallbladder functions as a reservoir for bile produced in your liver before the fluid drains into the duodenum.

Bile is produced continuously in your liver, even when your body isn't digesting food. Excess bile is turned into a more concentrated, potent solution in the gallbladder when some of the water that makes up bile is absorbed. When food passes into your duodenum, a hormone signals the gallbladder to release its stored bile.

The chemical breakdown of food in the digestive tract is most intensive in the duodenum. Here, digestive juices converge from the pancreas, liver and gallbladder and mix with juices secreted from the walls of the small intestine to carry out the breakdown. The duodenum, however, absorbs only small amounts of nutrients through the intestinal walls. Muscular contractions continue moving food waste through the digestive tract.

The next section of the small intestine, called the jejunum (je-JOO-num), is about 8 feet long. Here is where many nutrients are absorbed from food and passed into the bloodstream.

The final section of the small intestine, the ileum (IL-e-um), is about 12 feet long. Its primary duty is to absorb remaining nutrients from food waste. Absorption of vitamin B-12, an essential vitamin, occurs in the last few feet of the ileum, called the terminal ileum. Bile acids also are absorbed in the terminal ileum. When bile acids aren't removed, they pass into the large intestine and may cause diarrhea.

The journey of food through the small intestine generally takes between 30 minutes and three hours, depending on the composition of your meal.

Colon

The colon, also known as the large intestine, stores and removes any food waste that your body can't digest. The colon is shorter than the small intestine but its diameter is greater and almost completely frames your small intestine within the body. There are four sections of the colon: ascending, transverse, descending and sigmoid (see the illustration on page 23).

Food enters your colon through the ileocecal valve at the end of your small intestine. This muscular valve prevents food waste from returning to the ileum. By the time food residue reaches the colon, your body has absorbed nearly all of the nutrients it can.

What remains are water, electrolytes such as sodium and chloride, and waste products such as plant fiber, bacteria and dead cells shed from the lining of your digestive tract.

During the time that food waste passes through your colon, your body absorbs nearly all of the water from the waste. The remaining residue, called stool, is usually soft but formed. It's also loaded with bacteria, which are harmless to your body as long as your colon wall remains intact.

Problems by the numbers

The prevalence of digestive problems is reflected in these general statistics:

- More than 60 million Americans experience heartburn at least once a month. More than 15 million may have heartburn each day.

- About 50 million Americans have trouble digesting dairy products, a condition called lactose intolerance.

- An estimated 30 to 45 million Americans experience abdominal pain, gas, and diarrhea or constipation, associated with irritable bowel syndrome.

- More than 4 million Americans are bothered by frequent constipation.

- About 500,000 Americans develop a new peptic ulcer and about 4 million Americans experience a recurrence of peptic ulcers each year.

- About 3.2 million Americans are chronically infected with the hepatitis C virus.

- Cancer of the colon and rectum is second only to lung cancer as the leading cause of cancer-related deaths in the U.S. It takes more than 51,000 lives each year.

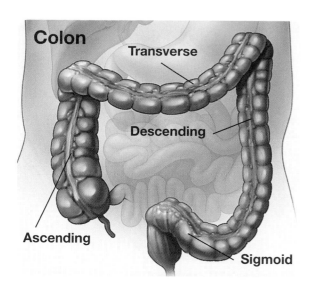

Colon

Transverse

Descending

Ascending

Sigmoid

These bacteria cause certain food products to ferment, producing gas. This gas, called flatus, is mainly an odorless mixture. The odors come from certain foods, especially those rich in sulfur, such as garlic and cabbage, or with sulfur-based preservatives such as bread, beer and potato chips.

As the food residue moves through your colon, muscle contractions separate and condense the waste into smaller segments. After each meal, considerable movement takes place in the descending colon, pushing the segments through your lower colon and into the rectum.

As your rectum begins to fill and stretch with waste, it signals your brain of the need to release stool. Sphincter muscles in your anus serve as a final valve. The

sphincter muscles relax as the muscles in your rectal walls contract to increase pressure and expel stool from your body. Sometimes, you need to exert additional pressure on the colon and rectum from your abdominal muscles.

Lifestyle issues

Are digestive problems more common today than they were years ago? There aren't any figures that provide a definitive answer. However, several indicators, including the popularity of over-the-counter medications, suggest this may be true. Some of the causes may be associated with your lifestyle.

Eating in a hurry
Hectic schedules have more people rushing through their meals or eating on the go. When you eat fast, you often overeat before your stomach can signal that it's full — which often leads to weight gain. You tend not to chew your food long enough or grind it into small enough pieces, forcing your digestive system to work harder.

When you gulp down food rapidly, you swallow more air than you would by eating slowly. This leads to belching and intestinal gas.

High-fat diet

Fast-food restaurants and prepackaged meals are popular conveniences today. But this type of diet often includes high fat and excess calories. The average American eats too much fat and not enough of the fiber found in fruits, vegetables and grains. Fiber helps food pass smoothly through your digestive tract. Fat does the opposite. It slows down digestion.

Studies also suggest that a diet high in saturated fats (animal fats) may increase your risk of cancer, especially colon cancer. Exactly how fat contributes to the development of cancer is unclear, but research suggests that it may promote the formation of cancer-causing substances (carcinogens).

Inactivity

Many people in the United States have increasingly sedentary lifestyles and don't participate in recreational sports or exercise. Regular physical activity is important for digestion because it helps speed the movement of food through your digestive tract in addition to helping you maintain a healthy weight.

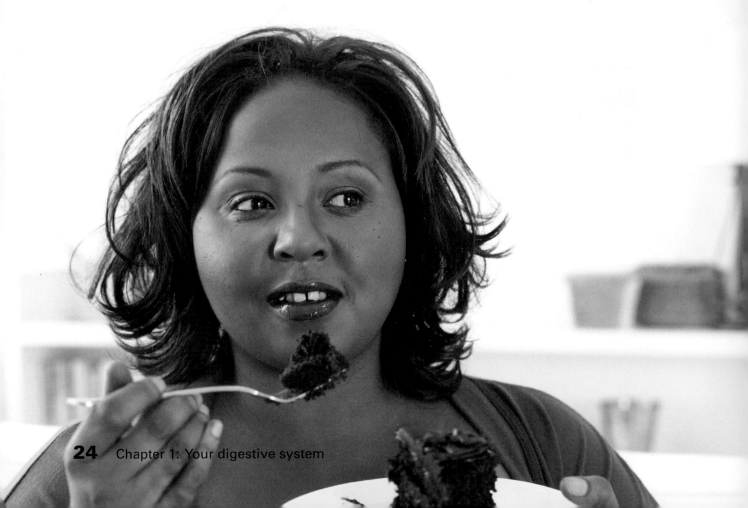

Obesity

A combination of too much fat in your diet and too little physical activity has resulted in a dramatic increase in the number of obese Americans. Over 30 percent of American adults have a body mass index (BMI) equal to or greater than 30. That means they're at least 30 percent above their healthy weight and are considered obese.

That figure represents more than a 50 percent jump in the rate of obesity from 1960, when about 13 percent of the adult population was obese.

Obesity is associated with a number of digestive problems. The most common is gastroesophageal reflux disease (GERD). The extra pounds increase the amount of pressure on your abdomen and stomach, which forces stomach acid to back up into your esophagus, causing heartburn and inflammation. Excess weight also increases your risk of gallbladder disease, and cancers of the esophagus, pancreas and colon.

Stress

Many Americans live stressful lives. When your body is focused on stress, you don't digest food as well. Stress reduces blood flow and affects muscle contractions in the digestive tract and the secretion of digestive juices.

Smoking

Smokers are more likely to have indigestion, stomach ulcers, active Crohn's disease and esophageal cancer. The good news is once you stop smoking tobacco, some of these digestive problems may disappear.

Alcohol

Consuming too much alcohol can:

- Inflame your stomach lining
- Relax the valve (lower esophageal sphincter) that seals and protects your esophagus from stomach acid
- Cause liver disease
- Cause pancreatitis

Women may be more susceptible to alcohol-related disorders because their bodies produce fewer enzymes to break down alcohol.

Over-the-counter medications

The overuse of many over-the-counter medications, including common nonsteroidal anti-inflammatory drugs (NSAIDs) such as aspirin, ibuprofen and naproxen sodium, can cause ulcers and gastrointestinal bleeding.

With these factors in mind, it should be clear that the health of your digestive tract has a lot to do with your lifestyle — the type of food you eat, how much food you eat, when you eat meals, how physically active you are, the type of exercise you do, the pace of your day and the amount of stress in your life.

Remarkably adaptive, the human digestive system can adjust to a wide variety of situations. It can also tolerate an astonishing amount of stress, as well as abuse from hurried or poorly planned meals. Over time, though, a poor diet, bad eating habits and inactivity may take their toll. Occasional symptoms, such as heartburn or abdominal pain, may eventually become more frequent and severe.

Not all digestive problems, however, stem from lifestyle. Some conditions are thought to be hereditary or related to an infection. For other digestive problems, there's no known cause.

Information in the following chapters provides the basics on some of the most common digestive conditions and helps you take care of your digestive system. It may help you prevent serious problems from developing or identify signs and symptoms and alert you on when to see your doctor.

Chapter 2

Recipe for healthy digestion

What you put on your plate has a lot to do with good digestion. But it's not only what you eat that's important. How much you eat, and the manner in which you eat — relaxed or hurried, focused or distracted — also play key roles. In other words, your daily food choices and the eating habits you regularly practice go a long way toward keeping your digestive system strong and healthy.

Of course, you can't prevent or manage all digestive problems simply by living a healthy lifestyle. Some digestive disorders are hereditary or occur for unknown reasons, and their treatment may require medical assistance. Still, there are many factors you can control and simple changes you can make to your lifestyle that may help.

For example, improving your diet with a variety of foods from different food groups, or taking moderate portions and not overeating, or eating sit-down meals at regular times — these are all simple changes that may have a significant impact on your digestive health.

If you stay committed, these changes turn into routine behaviors that last you for a lifetime. Success can be measured in many ways — you'll improve your digestive health, reduce your risk of disease, and look and feel better.

Think positive

Your best chance for successfully changing your lifestyle starts with a positive attitude. As you may be aware, knowing what you need to do and then actually doing it are two different things. After all, many people already know that a good diet and plenty of exercise are healthy — but that doesn't mean they're included in everyday life. Too often, your good intentions and best-laid plans are derailed by too much negative self-talk.

Self-talk — the internal dialogue you carry on with yourself each day — has a strong influence on the actions you take. When self-talk is negative, it tends to weaken your resolve and stall your progress. After all, if you can convince yourself that you can't cook, it seems reasonable to conclude, "Why even try to improve my diet if I'm so hopeless in the kitchen? I might as well continue eating just as I always have."

Examples of positive self-talk to counter that attitude include, "Well, I don't need to be a master chef to prepare a healthy meal" or "Even if I make a few mistakes at the beginning, I'll learn quickly and get better." A positive attitude can be the difference between successful change and giving up. It helps you challenge current beliefs, try different routines and adopt new ways of thinking. It carries you through periods of doubt. It gives you the confidence to know you can change.

A healthy diet

The food choices you make every day are starting points for better digestive health. It's important to eat a well-balanced diet that includes items from a variety of food groups.

Base your diet on the Mayo Clinic Healthy Weight Pyramid (see page 29) — a dietary guide that emphasizes balanced, health-promoting choices from six food groups. By following the pyramid recommendations for the types and amounts of food you eat, you also limit fat. Excess fat alters digestion and can lead to heartburn, bloating and constipation, in addition to increasing your weight, risk of heart disease, diabetes and perhaps colon cancer.

Vegetables and fruits: 7 to 10 servings

Vegetables and fruits share many attributes. In fact, some foods that we term vegetables, such as tomatoes, peppers and cucumbers, are technically fruits. Both food groups offer a wide array of flavors, textures and colors, providing sensory pleasure along with disease-fighting nutrients. The serving recommendations for vegetables and fruits are minimum amounts, unlike the recommendations for other food groups that set maximum limits.

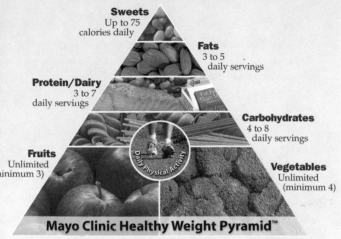

Sweets
Up to 75
calories daily

Fats
3 to 5
daily servings

Protein/Dairy
3 to 7
daily servings

Carbohydrates
4 to 8
daily servings

Daily physical activity

Fruits
Unlimited
(minimum 3)

Vegetables
Unlimited
(minimum 4)

Mayo Clinic Healthy Weight Pyramid™

The Mayo Clinic Healthy Weight Pyramid
is your tool for tracking and selecting healthy
foods. Number of servings is based on your
daily calorie goals — setting realistic goals
is explained on page 47 in the book.

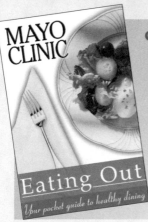

Vegetables and fruits are naturally low in calories and contain little or no fat. They provide beneficial fiber, vitamins, minerals and phytochemicals. Their location at the base of the pyramid indicates just how delicious and healthy vegetables and fruits are.

Fresh produce is best, but frozen varieties are good, too. Most canned vegetables are high in sodium — look for labels that indicate that no salt has been added, or rinse them before use. Look for labels on canned fruit that show the contents are canned in their own juices rather than in syrup. Dried fruits are high in fiber, but also in calories.

Carbohydrates: 4 to 8 servings
Carbohydrates include a wide range of foods that are major energy sources for your body. Most carbohydrates are plant based. They include grain products, such as breads, cereals, rice and pasta, and certain starchy vegetables, such as potatoes and corn. Along with vegetables and fruits, carbohydrates form the foundation of a healthy diet.

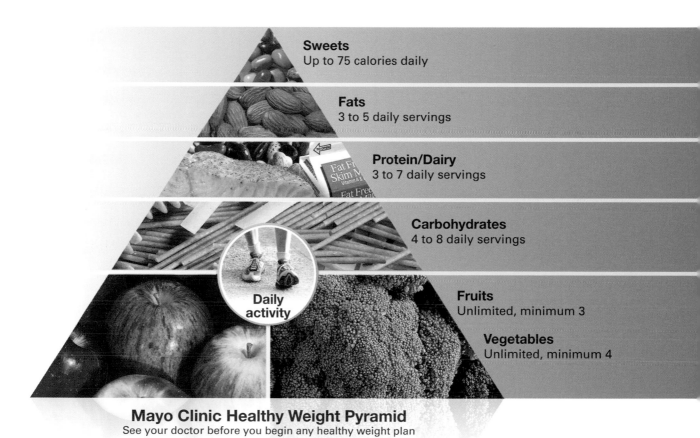

Sweets
Up to 75 calories daily

Fats
3 to 5 daily servings

Protein/Dairy
3 to 7 daily servings

Carbohydrates
4 to 8 daily servings

Daily activity

Fruits
Unlimited, minimum 3

Vegetables
Unlimited, minimum 4

Mayo Clinic Healthy Weight Pyramid
See your doctor before you begin any healthy weight plan

Sizing up a serving

The number of servings recommended for each food group may sound like a lot of food, but serving sizes may be smaller than you think. Here are some examples of what counts as one serving.

Food	Serving examples
Vegetables and fruits	1/2 cup (4 fl. oz.) 100 percent fruit juice 1 small orange, apple, banana or pear 2 cups raw leafy vegetables 1 cup cooked or chopped raw vegetables
Carbohydrates	1 slice whole-wheat bread 1/2 bagel or English muffin 1/3 to 1/2 cup cooked cereal, rice or pasta 1/2 to 3/4 cup ready-to-eat cereal 1/2 medium potato
Dairy products	1 cup (8 fl. oz.) low-fat or fat-free milk or yogurt 11/2 oz. natural cheese, such as cheddar 2/3 cup low-fat or fat-free cottage cheese
Poultry, fish, meat	2-3 oz. cooked skinless poultry, fish or lean meat
Legumes	1/2 cup cooked legumes (beans, dried peas or lentils)

Select products made with whole grains when possible. Whole grains are less processed and still contain their natural nutrients. Often when grains are processed, the bran and germ are stripped away, removing most of their vitamins and fiber. Generally, the less refined a carbohydrate food is, the better it is for you.

Protein and dairy: 3 to 7 servings

This group includes foods from both plant and animal sources. Protein-rich plant-based foods, including legumes such as beans, peas and lentils, are low in fat, cholesterol-free and excellent sources of fiber. Animal-based foods rich in protein, including fish and seafood, poultry, meat and eggs, are also sources of B vitamins, iron and zinc. However, many cuts of chicken, turkey, beef, lamb and pork can be high in saturated fat and cholesterol. Focus on lean cuts of meat, and remember to use the many other everyday foods that furnish protein as well.

Dairy products high in protein, including milk, yogurt and cheese, are outstanding sources of calcium and vitamin D — a vitamin that helps your body absorb calcium. Select low-fat or skim varieties. Some dairy products are high in fat and cholesterol, so low-fat or fat-free products are best.

Fats, sweets and alcohol: Sparingly

You need some fat in your diet but avoid saturated fats and trans fats. Make the healthier choices — olive oil, vegetable oils such as canola, and avocados, nuts and nut butters. All fats contain about the same number of calories, so even the healthier kinds should be used sparingly. Alcohol and sweets, such as candies and desserts, provide plenty of calories but little or no nutritional value. You don't have to give up these foods entirely, but be smart about your selections and portion sizes.

Eat fiber

Your digestive tract will accept almost any food you send its way. However, certain foods tend to pass more easily and quickly through your system and help it function properly. These foods are rich in dietary fiber, a nutrient that's an important part of a healthy diet and is especially important to digestion.

Plant foods — vegetables, fruits and foods made from whole grains — contain many vitamins and minerals that are essential for good health. They also contain compounds called phytochemicals that may protect against cancer and heart disease. Plant foods are also excellent sources of fiber.

Nutrition Facts

Serving Size 16 Crackers (31 g)
Servings Per Container About 9

Amount Per Serving

Calories 150   Calories from Fat 50

	% Daily Value*
Total Fat 6 g	9%
Saturated Fat 1g	6%
Trans Fat 0 g	
Polyunsaturated Fat 0 g	
Monounsaturated Fat 2 g	
Cholesterol 0 mg	0%
Sodium 270 mg	11%
Total Carbohydrate 21 mg	7%
Dietary Fiber 1 g	4%
Sugars 3 g	
Protein 2 g	

Vitamin A 0%	•	Vitamin C 0%	
Calcium 2%	•	Iron 6%	

* Percent Daily Values are based on a 2,000 calorie diet. Your daily values may be higher or lower depending on your calorie needs:

	Calories:	2,000	2,500

Packaged foods sold in the United States have a nutrition facts label. Nutrition facts are a quick guide to how a food fits into your eating plan.

In simple terms, fiber is the part of plant food that your body doesn't absorb — it's material that's indigestible and exits your body in stool. Fiber comes in two forms: soluble and insoluble, and fiber-rich foods usually contain both forms. Soluble fiber absorbs up to 15 times its weight in water as it moves through your digestive tract, producing softer stools. It's abundant in oats, barley, legumes and most fruits. Insoluble fiber, which is abundant in vegetables and whole grains, doesn't absorb water and gives stool its bulk.

The softening and bulking of stool helps prevent constipation and some types of diarrhea. This may also help relieve signs and symptoms of irritable bowel syndrome. These developments reduce pressure on the intestinal tract, lowering your risk of hemorrhoids and diverticular disease, a condition in which pouches form in intestinal walls that may become inflamed.

Fiber has other benefits. There's evidence that soluble fiber helps lower cholesterol and protect against cardiovascular disease. It does this by increasing the amount of bile — a substance your body produces to help digest fat — that's excreted in stool. To make more bile, your liver removes more cholesterol from your blood.

Fiber may also improve diabetes control by slowing digestion, thereby slowing the release of sugar into your bloodstream. However, it's uncertain whether this benefit comes from the fiber itself, or from other aspects of a high-fiber diet that may positively affect blood sugar control.

Where to find fiber

Depending on your age and sex, aim for 21 to 38 grams of fiber daily from a variety of food sources. To avoid digestive upset and gas that can come from eating too much fiber too quickly, gradually increase the amount you eat over a period of a couple of weeks. Here's the amount of fiber in some common foods.

Breads, cereals and other grain products	Grams		Grams
All-Bran Bran Buds, Kellogg's (1/2 cup)	20.0	Cheerios, General Mills (1 cup)	3.0
Fiber One, General Mills (1/2 cup)	14.0	Bread, Healthy Choice (1 slice)	3.0
100% Bran, Post (1/2 cup)	14.0	Shredded Wheat, Post (1 cup, bite size)	3.0
All-Bran Original, Kellogg's (1/2 cup)	10.0	Spaghetti, enriched (1 cup, cooked)	2.4
Grape Nuts, Post (1/2 cup)	7.0	Pumpernickel bread (1 slice)	2.1
Spaghetti, whole wheat (1 cup, cooked)	6.3	Egg noodles, enriched (1 cup, cooked)	1.9
Bagel, whole wheat (3 1/2 inch)	6.0	Whole-wheat bread (1 slice)	1.9
Cracklin' Oat Bran, Kellogg's (1/2 cup)	4.0	Cracked wheat bread (1 slice)	1.4
Raisin Bran, Post (1/2 cup)	4.0	Oatmeal bread (1 slice)	1.1
Oatmeal, quick/reg./inst. (1 cup, cooked)	4.0	Corn Flakes, Kellogg's (1 cup)	1.0
Rice, brown (1 cup, cooked)	3.5	White bread (1 slice)	0.6

Fruits			
Avocado (1 medium)	9.2	Orange (1 medium)	3.1
Raspberries (1 cup)	8.0	Banana (1 medium)	3.1
Prunes, dried (10)	6.7	Raisins, seedless (1/2 cup)	2.7
Dates, dried (10)	5.7	Grapefruit, pink & red (1/2 medium)	2.0
Pear, with skin (1 medium)	5.1	Peach (1 medium)	1.5
Blueberries (1 cup)	3.5	Cherries, sweet (10)	1.4
Apple, with skin (1 medium)	3.3	Applesauce, unsweetened (1/2 cup)	1.3
Strawberries (1 cup)	3.3		

Where to find fiber (cont.)

Legumes and vegetables (cooked, unless specified)

Food	Grams	Food	Grams
Beans, baked, homemade (1 cup)	13.9	Corn (1 cup)	3.9
Kidney beans, red (1 cup, boiled)	13.1	Popcorn, air-popped (3 cups)	3.6
Lima beans (1 cup)	9.0	Cauliflower (1 cup)	2.9
Peas, canned (1 cup)	8.3	Onions, raw (1 cup, chopped)	2.7
Squash, winter (1 cup, baked)	5.7	Potato, no skin (1 medium, boiled)	2.4
Broccoli (1 cup, boiled)	5.1	Carrots, raw (1 medium)	2.0
Sweet potato (1, baked with skin)	4.8	Cabbage, raw (1 cup, shredded)	1.8
Spinach (1 cup, boiled)	4.3	Tomato, raw (1 medium)	1.5
Green beans (1 cup)	4.0	Lettuce, iceberg (1 cup, chopped)	0.7
Chunky vegetable soup, Campbell's (1 cup)	4.0	Celery, raw (1 stalk, 7 1/2" long)	0.6

Cooking ingredients

Food	Grams	Food	Grams
Corn bran (1/3 cup)	19.8	Oat bran, uncooked (1/3 cup)	4.8
Flour, whole wheat (1 cup)	14.6	Wheat germ, crude (1/4 cup)	3.8
Soy flour, low-fat (1 cup)	14.1	Flour, white (1 cup)	3.4
Cornmeal, white, enriched (1 cup)	6.4	Graham cracker crumbs (1/2 cup)	2.6

Adapted from: USDA National Nutrient Database
for Standard Reference, Release 22, 2009

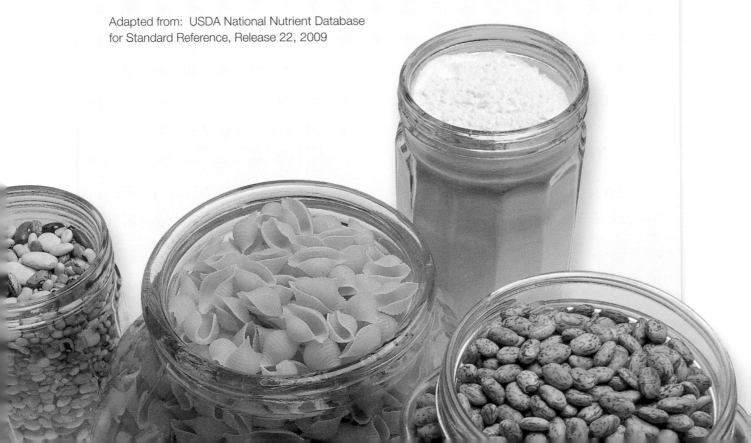

The benefits of fiber with regard to cancer remain unclear. Despite the lack of conclusive evidence, the scientific consensus is that dietary fiber protects against colon cancer. It's also possible that other components in high-fiber foods, such as phytochemicals, may have roles as protective agents.

Unfortunately, most of us don't get enough fiber. Americans typically consume 12 to 18 grams of fiber daily. Dietary guidelines recommend two to three times that amount. For adults 50 years and younger, the recommendation is 38 grams of fiber a day for men and 25 grams for women. For adults over 50, it's 30 grams for men and 21 grams for women.

Drink plenty of fluids

Fluids help dissolve nutrients in the food you eat, making them easier to absorb. Fluids lubricate food waste so that it passes more easily through your digestive tract. Fluids also soften stool, helping to prevent constipation. Every day, you replace fluids lost through urine and bowel movements (in addition to other types of fluids that you lose through breathing and perspiration), which allows your body systems to continue functioning properly.

Drinking water is generally the best way to replace fluid. Milk, juices and other beverages are about 90 percent water, so they also can help meet your daily fluid needs (see sidebar below for more information). Caffeinated beverages and alcohol generally don't count. In some people, they act as diuretics, increasing urination and fluid loss. Caffeine and alcohol may also contribute to heartburn and indigestion.

In the morning, a warm beverage may be preferable to a cold one, especially if you're bothered by constipation. About 30 minutes after drinking warm liquid, your body may have a natural urge to pass stool. For some, drinking a caffeinated beverage also may stimulate a bowel movement.

How much is enough?
To determine the amount of fluid your body needs each day, divide your weight (in pounds) in half. The answer is the approximate amount of fluid (in ounces) recommended daily. For most people, the figure equates to at least eight 8-ounce glasses.

Practice good eating habits

How you eat can be just as important for good digestion as what you eat. Poor digestion may simply be due to the bad habits you practice during or between meals.

Eat moderate proportions
Large meals put increased demands on digestion, and your body is able to produce only a certain amount of digestive juices in order to meet those demands. Large amounts of food also increase the amount of waste moving through your digestive tract, which may lead to bloating. Moderate portions, on the other hand, are digested more comfortably and reduce the risk of overeating.

Eat at regular times
Your digestive organs operate best when you follow a regular schedule. People who eat whenever they feel like it tend to eat less nutritious foods than those who eat three meals a day. With a regular schedule, your digestive system has time to rest between meals. Skipping meals leads to excessive hunger, which often results in overeating.

Eat in the morning
The morning is one of the best times of day to take advantage of regular muscle contractions taking place in your colon (gastrocolic reflex). This reflex helps move waste from the colon to the rectum, triggering an urge to expel stool. Eating breakfast loads your digestive system with food — and ultimately food waste — helping to promote regular bowel movements.

Relax while you eat
Your state of mind while you eat also can affect your digestion. When you're relaxed, you tend to chew your food more completely, gastric and intestinal juices flow more freely, and digestive muscles contract and relax normally. When you eat too fast, you don't chew food thoroughly and often swallow air, causing belching or bloating. Eating when you feel stressed interferes with normal functioning of your intestines, and can result in stomach upset, heartburn, constipation or diarrhea.

Maintain a healthy weight

Digestive problems can occur no matter what your weight. But heartburn, bloating and constipation tend to be more common in people who are overweight, perhaps because they tend to exercise less and eat more fat and less fiber. Maintaining a healthy weight can often help prevent or reduce these problems.

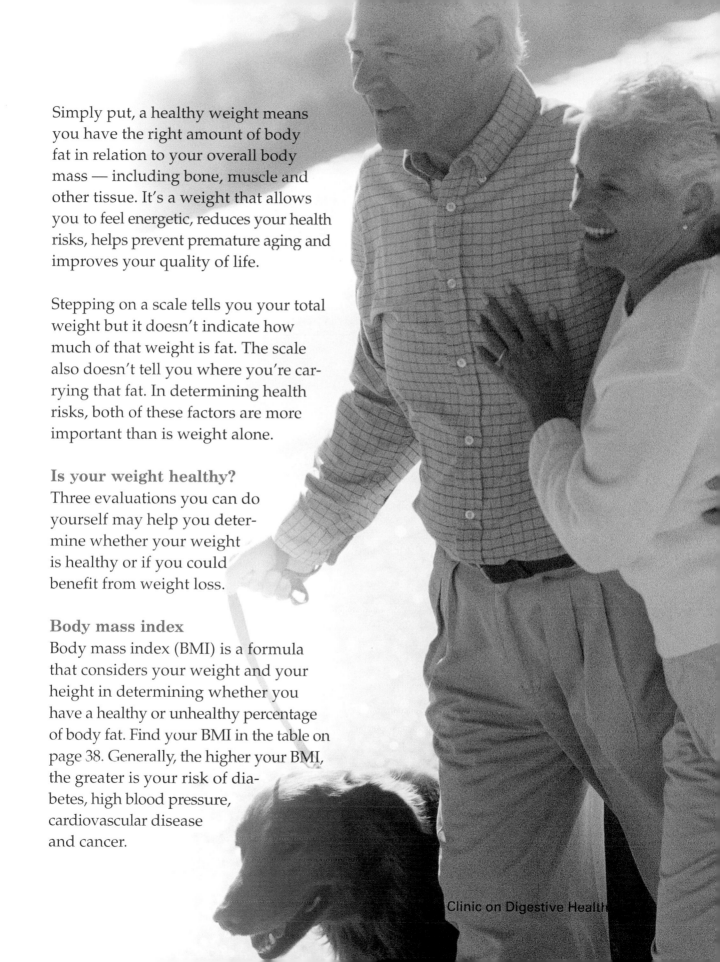

Simply put, a healthy weight means you have the right amount of body fat in relation to your overall body mass — including bone, muscle and other tissue. It's a weight that allows you to feel energetic, reduces your health risks, helps prevent premature aging and improves your quality of life.

Stepping on a scale tells you your total weight but it doesn't indicate how much of that weight is fat. The scale also doesn't tell you where you're carrying that fat. In determining health risks, both of these factors are more important than is weight alone.

Is your weight healthy?

Three evaluations you can do yourself may help you determine whether your weight is healthy or if you could benefit from weight loss.

Body mass index

Body mass index (BMI) is a formula that considers your weight and your height in determining whether you have a healthy or unhealthy percentage of body fat. Find your BMI in the table on page 38. Generally, the higher your BMI, the greater is your risk of diabetes, high blood pressure, cardiovascular disease and cancer.

Clinic on Digestive Health

To determine your body mass index, locate your height in the left column and follow the row across until you reach the weight nearest yours. Look at the top of the column for your BMI number. If your weight is slightly more or slightly less than the weight shown in the column, your BMI may be correspondingly slightly more or slightly less.

A BMI of 19 to 24.9 is considered healthy. A BMI of 25 to 29.9 signifies being overweight, and a BMI of 30 or more indicates obesity. If your BMI

What's your BMI?

	Normal		Overweight					Obese				
BMI	19	24	25	26	27	28	29	30	35	40	45	50
Height						Weight in pounds						
4'10"	91	115	119	124	129	134	138	143	167	191	215	239
4'11"	94	119	124	128	133	138	143	148	173	198	222	247
5'0"	97	123	128	133	138	143	148	153	179	204	230	255
5'1"	100	127	132	137	143	148	153	158	185	211	238	264
5'2"	104	131	136	142	147	153	158	164	191	218	246	273
5'3"	107	135	141	146	152	158	163	169	197	225	254	282
5'4"	110	140	145	151	157	163	169	174	204	232	262	291
5'5"	114	144	150	156	162	168	174	180	210	240	270	300
5'6"	118	148	155	161	167	173	179	186	216	247	278	309
5'7"	121	153	159	166	172	178	185	191	223	255	287	319
5'8"	125	158	164	171	177	184	190	197	230	262	295	328
5'9"	128	162	169	176	182	189	196	203	236	270	304	338
5'10"	132	167	174	181	188	195	202	209	243	278	313	348
5'11"	136	172	179	186	193	200	208	215	250	286	322	358
6'0"	140	177	184	191	199	206	213	221	258	294	331	368
6'1"	144	182	189	197	204	212	219	227	265	302	340	378
6'2"	148	186	194	202	210	218	225	233	272	311	350	389
6'3"	152	192	200	208	216	224	232	240	279	319	359	399
6'4"	156	197	205	213	221	230	238	246	287	328	369	410

Source: National Institutes of Health (NIH), 1998

*Asians with a BMI of 23 or higher may have an increased risk of health problems.

is less than 18.5, you're underweight, which may put you at increased risk of health problems.

Waist circumference

Medical conditions associated with excess weight, such as high blood pressure, high cholesterol, coronary artery disease, stroke and diabetes, are influenced by the locations where fat is stored on your body.

People who carry most of their weight around their waists are referred to as apple shaped. The fat located in and around their abdominal organs increases the risk of disease. People who carry most of their weight around their hips and thighs are referred to as pear shaped. Their risks aren't as high.

To determine whether you're carrying too much weight around your middle, measure your waist circumference just above your hipbones, usually at the level of your navel. A measurement exceeding 40 inches (102 centimeters) in men and 35 inches (89 centimeters) in women indicates an apple shape and increased health risks, especially if you have a BMI of 25 or higher.

Medical history

An evaluation of your medical history, along with that of your family, is a third factor in determining whether you have a healthy weight. Ask yourself the following questions:

- Do you have a health condition, such as high blood pressure, heart disease, type 2 diabetes or fatty liver (steatosis), that would benefit from weight loss?
- Do you have a family history of a weight-related illness, such as cardiovascular disease, diabetes, high blood pressure or colon or breast cancer?
- Have you gained considerable weight since high school? Weight gain in adulthood is associated with increased health risks.
- Do you smoke cigarettes, have more than two alcoholic drinks a day or live with considerable stress? In combination with these behaviors, excess weight can have greater health implications.

Do you need to lose weight?

If your BMI indicates that you aren't overweight, if you're not carrying too much weight around your abdomen, and if you answered no to all of the medical history questions, you're probably at a healthy weight and there's little advantage to changing your weight.

Foods high in fat

The following products are generally loaded with fat. Some you may avoid entirely and the others, use in moderation.

- Pastries, doughnuts, cakes, cookies, sweet rolls and pies
- Most crackers
- Most chips (potato chips, corn chips)
- Cheeses (other than cheeses made from skim milk)
- Nuts, peanuts, peanut butter
- Cooking oils
- Margarine, butter, lard and shortening
- Cream and ice cream
- Fried foods
- Hot dogs and luncheon meats

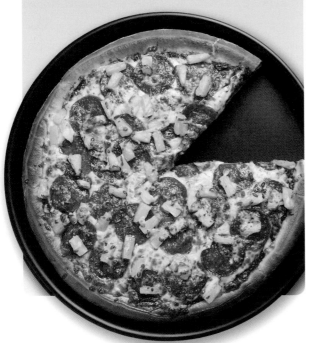

If your BMI is between 25 and 30 or your waist measurement exceeds the healthy guidelines, and you answered yes to one or more of the medical history questions, you'll probably benefit from losing a few pounds. Discuss weight concerns with your doctor at your next checkup.

If your BMI is 30 or more, losing weight is recommended to improve your health and help reduce your risk of weight-related illness. Discuss the next steps you should take with your doctor.

If you need to lose weight

Many products and programs promise to help you shed pounds, but they aren't always safe or effective. Too often, you gain back the weight you initially lost. A better approach to weight loss may be with permanent lifestyle changes. The following guidelines may help you be successful.

Make a commitment
Only you can help yourself lose weight — your motivation comes because it's something you want to do, not what someone else wants you to do. However, that doesn't mean that you have to act alone. You can look to others when you need support and encouragement.

Think positively

Don't dwell on what you're giving up in order to lose weight. Instead, concentrate on what you're gaining.

Get your priorities straight

Timing is crucial to success. Don't try to lose weight while you're distracted by other problems. If you're having financial troubles, or a friend or family member is ill, it may not be the best time to focus on a weight program.

Set realistic goals

Don't aim for an unrealistic weight that's based on the social ideals of thinness. Instead, try for a comfortable weight that you maintained as a young adult. If you've always been overweight, aim for a weight that improves your signs and symptoms and raises your energy level. Even modest weight loss — about 10 percent of your body weight — has health benefits.

Accept the fact that healthy weight loss is slow and steady. A good weight-loss plan generally involves losing no more than 1 to 2 pounds a week.

Know your habits

Chances are, many behaviors you feel you were born with are actually ones you've learned how to do over time. Factors such as emotions, self-image, social pressure, stress and lack of awareness have very little to do with your stomach but strongly influence what you eat and how you eat.

It's good to know that if a behavior can be learned, it can also be unlearned. Take stock of your behaviors and try to identify factors that may be the cause of unhealthy, hard-to-break eating habits. Changing behavior varies from person to person, but identifying the cause is an important step in making it happen.

Don't starve yourself

Losing weight should not involve damaging your health. Cutting calories to fewer than 1,200 if you're a woman or 1,400 if you're a man makes it harder to get enough of certain nutrients your body needs to stay healthy. It also promotes temporary loss of fluids and a loss of healthy muscle, instead of a permanent loss of fat. Eating too few calories doesn't satisfy your hunger until the next meal, which leads to between-meal snacking.

Liquid meals, diet pills and special food combinations aren't the answer to long-term weight control and better health. The best way to lose weight is to eat more nutritious foods — vegetables, fruits, whole grains — and fewer foods that contain fat and sugar.

Calories burned in 1 hour

The calories you burn for a variety of activities varies widely depending on the type of exercise, intensity level and individual.

Activity (one-hour duration)	Weight of person and calories burned		
	160 pounds (73 kilograms)	200 pounds (91 kilograms)	240 pounds (109 kilograms)
Aerobics, low impact	365	455	545
Aerobics, water	292	364	436
Basketball game	584	728	872
Bicycling, < 10 mph, leisure	292	364	436
Bowling	219	273	327
Dancing, ballroom	219	273	327
Football, touch, flag, general	584	728	872
Golfing, carrying clubs	329	410	491
Hiking	438	546	654
Ice skating	511	637	763
Jogging, 5 mph	584	728	872
Racquetball, casual, general	511	637	763
Rope jumping	730	910	1,090
Rowing, stationary	511	637	763
Running, 8 mph	986	1,229	1,472
Skiing, cross-country	511	637	763
Skiing, downhill	365	455	545
Softball or baseball	365	455	545
Stair treadmill	657	819	981
Swimming, laps	511	637	763
Tennis, singles	584	728	872
Volleyball	292	364	436
Walking, 2 mph	183	228	273
Walking, 3.5 mph	277	346	414
Weightlifting	219	273	327

Based on Ainsworth BE, et al., Medicine & Science in Sports & Exercise, 2000

Increase your activity

Eating provides you with calories. Physical activity burns off those calories. And the more physically active you are, the more calories you burn. Exercise is the single most important factor in successfully managing your weight over the long-term. In addition to weight control, physical activity offers many health benefits.

Stay committed

Don't let occasional setbacks — and there will be some — weaken your commitment. If you find yourself falling back into former bad habits, return to the strategies you followed in the first place to lose weight. It's not enough to eat nutritious foods and exercise for a few weeks or months. You need to make new, beneficial behaviors a permanent part of your life.

Weight-loss medications and surgery

Medications may be used as tools to help make changes in your diet, but they are often not the solution to your weight problem. Prescription medications for weight loss may be appropriate for moderately overweight and obese people with health complications related to weight. It's best if the individuals using these drugs are enrolled in a weight management program.

Generally, surgery for weight loss is reserved for people who are severely obese and who have health problems as a result. Direct questions about medications and surgery to your doctor.

Get regular exercise

Physical activity is any movement you do that burns calories — from gardening to cleaning the house to taking a break from your office desk. Exercise is a structured, repetitive form of physical activity — such as swimming laps, bicycling, brisk walking and lifting weights. All physical activity you do throughout the day can be good for you, even if it's not a form of exercise.

It's been said that the best form of physical activity is the one you'll do, and the best time to do it is whenever you can. That's a good place to start. But check with your doctor before starting any exercise program, particularly if you're middle-aged or older, are significantly overweight, or have been inactive for several years. Your doctor can help you choose activities that are safe and appropriate for you.

Aerobic exercise — exercise that increases your breathing and heart rate — is the most beneficial for healthy

Before you get started

It's often a good idea to talk with your doctor before starting an exercise program. If you have a health problem or you're at risk of heart disease, you may need to take some precautions while you exercise. It's essential that you see your doctor if you:

- Are unsure of your health status
- Have experienced chest discomfort, shortness of breath or dizziness during or right after exercise or strenuous activity
- Are a man age 40 years or older, or a woman age 50 years or older, and haven't had a recent physical examination
- Have a blood pressure of 140/90 millimeters of mercury or higher
- Have diabetes, heart, lung or kidney disease, or are obese
- Have a family history of heart-related problems before age 55
- Are taking medication for diabetes, high blood pressure, heart problems or another medical condition
- Have bone or joint problems that could be made worse by some forms of physical activity

digestion. In addition to improving the health of your heart and lungs, aerobic exercise stimulates the activity of your stomach and intestinal muscles, helping to move food and waste through your digestive tract.

Aerobic exercise also builds stamina, helps to strengthen your immune system, and promotes weight loss. The table on page 42 shows how many calories you can burn from doing a variety of different physical activities — some may appeal to you.

Remember that you don't have to do all of your exercising at one time. Doing 20 minutes of walking during the morning, 25 minutes of lawn mowing in the afternoon and perhaps 15 minutes of bicycling in the evening all count toward keeping fit. The following are tips for building an exercise program.

Walk before you run
Over enthusiasm may lead you to the "terrible toos" of exercise — too much, too hard, too often, too soon. This

all-or-nothing approach is a recipe for discouragement, not to mention injury. Start slowly and gradually build up.

Do what you enjoy

If you want an exercise program that you'll stay with, the program should be filled with activities that are fun for you. Many different types of activity can increase your fitness level. The trick is choosing ones that also stimulate and entertain you.

Pick a time and stick with it

Schedule specific times to exercise, whether it's a two-hour workout or at short, regular intervals. Don't try to exercise in your "spare time." If you don't make it a priority, exercise will be pushed aside for other concerns.

Warm up

Give yourself time to warm up before exercise with easy walking and gentle stretching. Then speed up activity to a pace you can continue without getting overly tired. Also, allow time to cool down after exercise.

Listen to your body

Exercise shouldn't cause discomfort. If you feel pain, shortness of breath, dizziness or nausea, take a break — you may be pushing yourself too hard. If you're not feeling well, take a day or two off and resume as soon as you can.

Aerobic exercise

Following physician approval, try to do 30 to 60 minutes of aerobic activity most, if not all, days of the week. Walking is the most common aerobic activity because it's easy, convenient and inexpensive. All you need is a good pair of walking shoes. Other aerobic exercises include bicycling, basketball, golfing (walking, not riding), social dancing, volleyball, aerobic dancing, hiking, jogging, skiing, running, tennis and swimming.

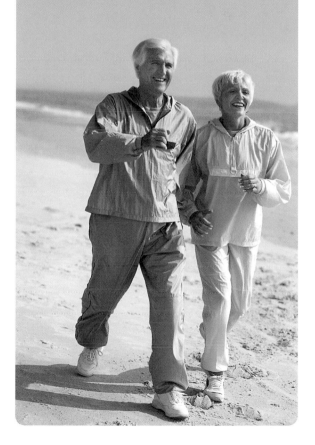

Use realistic strategies

If you aren't a morning person, setting the alarm clock for 4:30 a.m. to get up and exercise isn't going to work. Try to exercise after work. If your knees can't handle jogging, try cycling or swimming.

Control stress

Digestive problems can occur for reasons other than a poor diet or lack of exercise. Your digestive tract is long and complex, and many lifestyle factors can influence how well it functions. One of the most influential factors is stress.

Everyone experiences stress. What's important is to recognize when you're feeling stressed, and to take steps to relieve tension with exercise or relaxation techniques. Left untreated, stress can take a toll on your health, cause weight gain, create sleep troubles and negatively affect your digestion.

When you're under stress, your body reacts as if you're in danger. It pumps extra blood to your muscles so you'll have more energy either to fight off an attack or to run away. This leaves less blood volume to support digestion. Your digestive muscles exert less effort, your body secretes smaller amounts of the compounds that aid digestion (enzymes), and the passage of food and waste through your digestive tract shifts into low gear. This produces symptoms such as heartburn, bloating and constipation.

Sometimes stress does the opposite. It speeds passage of food through your intestines, causing abdominal pain and diarrhea. Stress may also worsen symptoms of digestive conditions such as ulcers, irritable bowel syndrome and ulcerative colitis.

Regular physical activity is one way to help you reduce and manage the stress in your life. Exercise often serves as a sort of timeout from problems — you tend to focus on the immediate task at hand and not on the tensions of the day. As you exert your body, your mind senses a feeling of calm and control.

Limit alcohol

There's evidence that some alcoholic beverages may benefit your health, especially in reducing your risk of heart disease. Regardless, limit alcohol to moderate amounts — no more than one drink a day for women or two drinks a day for men, and just one drink a day if you're over 65, whether you're female or male. A drink is defined as 12 ounces of beer, 5 ounces of wine, or 1.5 ounces of 80-proof distilled spirits.

Too much alcohol — anything above a moderate amount — can cause digestive disorders. Alcohol may inflame the stomach lining and relax the valve preventing stomach acid from backing up into your esophagus. This can increase your risk of bleeding or heartburn.

Alcohol may also aggravate symptoms such as diarrhea or nausea. Excessive alcohol is a leading cause of liver and pancreatic disease. When combined with tobacco, alcohol greatly increases your risk of mouth and esophageal cancers.

Avoid tobacco

If you chew or smoke tobacco, you may be more likely to experience heartburn. That's because nicotine in tobacco may increase stomach acid production and decrease the production of sodium bicarbonate, a fluid that neutralizes stomach acid. Air swallowed during smoking can produce belching or bloating from gas. In addition, smoking puts you at increased risk of peptic ulcers and cancers of the mouth, throat and esophagus.

Use medications cautiously

Almost all medications affect digestion in one way or another. Often the effects are mild and go unnoticed, but some drugs produce signs and symptoms, especially if you take them regularly. For example, narcotics taken to relieve pain can produce constipation, medications taken for high blood pressure can cause diarrhea or constipation, and antibiotics taken to fight infection can cause nausea or diarrhea.

Some of the most potentially damaging medications, however, are nonsteroidal anti-inflammatory drugs (NSAIDs). These medications include the over-the-counter drugs aspirin, ibuprofen (Advil, Motrin, others), naproxen (Aleve) and ketoprofen.

When taken occasionally and as directed, NSAIDs are generally safe. When taken regularly, or if you take more than the recommended amounts, NSAIDs may cause nausea, stomach pain, stomach bleeding or ulcers.

That's because NSAIDs inhibit production of an enzyme called cyclooxygenase (cox). This enzyme produces hormone-like substances called prostaglandins that trigger inflammation and pain. However, prostaglandins also have a beneficial effect. They help protect your stomach lining against harmful acid.

If you take an NSAID regularly, talk with your doctor about ways to limit the drug's side effects, including taking the medication with food.

A newer class of medications called COX-2 inhibitors are generally less damaging to your digestive system than are NSAIDs. Unlike NSAIDs, these medications interfere mainly with the production of prostaglandins associated with inflammation and pain, and less with those substances that are involved in digestion.

Some studies have shown COX-2 inhibitors relieve joint pain with fewer side effects than traditional NSAIDs. However, more recent studies have found an increased risk of cardiovascular problems, including heart attack and stroke,

in some people who used COX-2 inhibitors long-term. Other serious but rare side effects of this class of medication may include stomach or intestinal bleeding, kidney or liver problems and allergic reactions.

Chapter 3

Gut feelings

You know the feeling. You've had it before, and you'll most likely have it again. It may be an uneasy sense of nausea or an attack of diarrhea urging you to the nearest bathroom. Perhaps it's that all too familiar sear of heartburn after a heavy meal.

Almost everyone occasionally experiences signs and symptoms that suggest something is not quite right in his or her digestive tract.

Often, two or more signs and symptoms occur at the same time, making it hard to describe exactly what the feeling is. When you complain of "indigestion," for example, you may actually be referring to a range of signs and symptoms, such as bloating, belching, nausea and mild cramping.

It's also not always clear what's causing your problem. There are many complex organs, functions and interconnections in your digestive tract. Certain signs and symptoms will almost always signal a digestive disorder of some kind — for example, if you have difficulty swallowing, diarrhea or constipation — but other signs and symptoms may, in fact, be more general in nature. This would include nausea, intestinal gas, abdominal pain and loss of appetite.

More often than not, there's little to worry about with occasional digestive problems other than minor discomfort. They're often temporary and possible to relieve with self-care. And sometimes, the problems are caused by things you do — which may give you some control over fixing them.

Behaviors that frequently cause digestive problems include:

- Eating spicy foods or fatty foods
- Eating too much
- Eating too fast
- Drinking too much caffeine or alcohol
- Smoking tobacco
- Experiencing stress or anxiety

How much discomfort you feel from any one of these behaviors is difficult to gauge — some people may be affected a lot, while others are affected very little or not at all. Typically, your signs and symptoms start to diminish soon after you stop doing whatever it is that triggered the problem, and they gradually disappear after a few hours.

It's when digestive signs and symptoms persist or worsen over days or even weeks that you have more reason to be concerned. They could signal a condition that deserves medical attention. Whenever the problems are making a noticeable impact on your quality of life, don't hesitate to discuss your concerns with your doctor.

This chapter may help you better understand the most common digestive signs and symptoms, and what may — or may not — be producing them. But this knowledge alone is not enough to resolve your problem. If you become concerned, it's important to see your doctor. Together, you may be able to identify a cause. A physical examination, along with questions about your

Common reasons for a doctor visit

Many digestive complaints can prompt people to schedule medical visits. Some of the most common are discussed in this chapter:

- Difficulty swallowing
- Chest pain and heartburn
- Belching, bloating and intestinal gas
- Indigestion

- Nausea and vomiting
- Abdominal pain
- Diarrhea or constipation
- Bleeding
- Weight loss

specific signs and symptoms, eating and exercise habits and daily routine, may be all that's necessary to allay your worries. Further testing (described in Chapter 4) may be necessary to explore more-serious problems.

Difficulty swallowing

Most people take swallowing for granted. They take a bite of food, chew, swallow and don't give it a second thought. For other people, difficulty with swallowing can be a daily problem.

If you get the feeling when you swallow that food is sticking in your throat or chest, you may have dysphagia (dis-FAY-jee-uh). The term comes from the Greek words *dys* (difficult) and *phagia* (to eat). Dysphagia can occur in two locations.

Pharynx

The pharynx is at the back of the throat and leads into your esophagus. If you have pharyngeal dysphagia, you have trouble moving food from your mouth and throat into your upper esophagus. The problem often but not always stems from weakened throat muscles because of a stroke or a neuromuscular disorder, such as muscular dystrophy or Parkinson's disease. Other signs and symptoms may include choking or coughing while swallowing, regurgitating fluid (or sometimes food) through the nose, a weak voice and weight loss.

Esophagus

Esophageal dysphagia refers to the sensation of food sticking or getting hung up in your esophagus. This form is more common than pharyngeal dysphagia, and is often accompanied by pressure or pain in your chest. Other signs and symptoms may include:

- Painful swallowing
- Sore throat
- Persistent cough
- Gurgling sounds

There are many reasons for esophageal dysphagia. One of the most common is a narrowing of the lower esophagus due to the formation of scar tissue.

The scar tissue is caused by stomach acid backing up into the esophagus and inflaming tissue (gastroesophageal reflux disease, or GERD). Inflammation of the lower esophagus may also occur that is secondary to GERD or infection, causing dysphagia.

Dysphagia can be the result of tumors (noncancerous or cancerous), radiation burns from cancer treatment, or formation of Schatzki's ring — a band of tissue that narrows the lower esophagus. In addition, the esophageal muscles that propel food to your stomach can weaken with age, making it more difficult to swallow. Diseases such as achalasia or scleroderma can weaken esophageal muscles.

One other possible cause of dysphagia is a diverticulum, a small pouch that can form in the back of your pharynx, just above the esophagus. Food particles may enter and fill the pouch, pressing it against the upper esophagus and interfering with swallowing. The food particles may be regurgitated, producing gurgling sounds and bad breath. They may also travel into your lungs, causing a cough and sometimes difficult breathing.

An occasional episode of swallowing difficulty typically isn't a serious problem, and may simply stem from not chewing your food well enough or eating too fast. But if the episodes are frequent or your symptoms are severe, see your doctor.

Treating dysphagia

How dysphagia may be treated will depend on its cause.

Physical therapy
If your swallowing difficulty is a result of weakened muscles in the esophagus, a physical therapist may assist you with techniques that help you swallow better.

Drug therapy
For dysphagia stemming from GERD, prescription medications are often effective in preventing the reflux of stomach acid into the esophagus. For dysphagia associated with infection or inflammation, medications may also be helpful.

Tissue stretching
If your esophagus is narrowed by scar tissue, hindering the passage of food, your doctor may use a device to stretch (dilate) the tissue, threading it through a slender, flexible tube (endoscope) that's been inserted down your esophagus. Often, the device is a deflated balloon that's placed in the narrowed section and then inflated to widen the passageway.

Surgery
In case of a tumor or a diverticulum, surgery is often necessary to clear the esophagus.

Modified diet

Sometimes it's necessary to modify the consistency of your diet until a cause of the problem is diagnosed and treated. Depending on the type and extent of your dysphagia, you may need to limit your diet to soft, puréed or liquid foods.

» *To learn more*

For additional information on conditions that may cause swallowing difficulty see these chapters.
Chapter 5: Gastroesophageal reflux disease (GERD)
Chapter 14: Cancer

Chest pain and heartburn

Chest pain can occur for any number of reasons: Warning sign of heart attack, lack of oxygen to your heart muscle (angina pectoris), a lung condition or inflammation of rib cage cartilage.

Many times, though, chest pain isn't heart or lung related. Rather, it stems from a digestive problem. For example, the pain associated with inflamma-

tion in your gallbladder (a gallbladder attack) can spread to your chest. The most common type of digestive-related chest pain, however, is associated with what many people know as heartburn.

Heartburn is a term describing a burning sensation in your chest that may start in your upper abdomen and radiate all the way up into your neck. Heartburn isn't a disease. Rather, it's a symptom. At times, especially when you're lying down, heartburn can be associated with a sour taste in your mouth — caused by stomach acid that backs up into your upper esophagus and mouth.

Normally, stomach acid stays in your stomach, kept there by the lower esophageal sphincter. This ring of muscle functions as a valve, opening only when you swallow, belch or vomit. But sometimes the valve relaxes or weakens, allowing stomach acid to regurgitate into your esophagus, producing a burning sensation.

Many infants are born with an immature sphincter valve, which is why they often spit up milk or food. By age 1, the valve is more fully developed and the flowing back (reflux) of stomach acid into their esophagus becomes much less common.

Among adults, occasional bouts of heartburn are common and can occur for many reasons — although an exact cause may never be found for some people. Being overweight, overeating, or lying down too soon after a meal puts pressure on the sphincter valve, and may cause it to open slightly. Through the small opening, stomach acid flows into the esophagus. Too much alcohol or caffeine, or certain foods also can relax the sphincter or increase production of stomach acid.

If you have heartburn several times a week or you need to take antacids frequently, see your doctor. Your heartburn may be a symptom of a more serious condition, such as GERD. If your heartburn seems to be getting worse or is different from normal — especially if it's accompanied by radiating pain in an arm — seek medical help immediately. Instead of heartburn, your pain may be the warning of a heart attack.

» *To learn more*

For additional information on conditions that may produce heartburn or chest pain see these chapters.
Chapter 5: Gastroesophageal reflux disease (GERD)
Chapter 11: Gallstones

Belching, bloating and intestinal gas

A buildup of air and gas in your digestive tract is a natural part of the digestive process. When you swallow food, you often swallow air with it that remains in your stomach and intestines for awhile. Food residue in your colon is another source of gas formation as the bacteria that naturally reside in your colon begin to ferment the undigested food particles.

It's natural to experience occasional discomfort when air or gas builds up in your digestive tract and to expel the air or gas as a way to relieve the problem. However, some people frequently complain of having "too much gas" in their systems. Their complaints usually involve one of three forms of distress: excessive belching, bloating or passing gas from the rectum (flatulence).

Belching

Belching, or burping, is a way for your body to expel excess air that you swallow while eating or drinking. This buildup can happen from eating too fast, talking while you eat or drinking carbonated beverages.

When you belch, air that has built up in your stomach is forced up into your esophagus and out of your mouth. An occasional belch is normal to relieve stomach fullness, but if you belch frequently, it may be a simple fact that you're swallowing too much air. Some people who belch repeatedly — even when they're not eating or drinking — are swallowing air as a nervous habit.

Belching also can result from the reflux of stomach acid into your esophagus. You may swallow frequently to clear the acid, which leads to more air intake and further belching.

Naturally, the best way to reduce belching is to swallow less air. These suggestions also may help.

Eat and drink slowly
Typically, the more time you take to eat and drink, the less air you swallow.

Drink fewer carbonated beverages
Soft drinks and beer release carbon dioxide gas, increasing the volume of air in your digestive system.

Avoid gum and hard candy
When you suck on hard candy or chew gum, you swallow more often than you normally would. Part of what you're swallowing is air.

Don't use a straw
You swallow more air sucking on a straw than you do sipping from a glass.

Don't smoke
When you inhale the smoke from tobacco products, you also inhale and swallow air.

Check your dentures
Loosefitting dentures can cause you to swallow excess air while you're drinking or eating.

If these steps don't help reduce excess air in your stomach, see your doctor to rule out more-serious conditions associated with belching, such as GERD or stomach inflammation (gastritis).

Bloating

Bloating is a common term for the buildup of gas in your stomach and intestines. Many times, bloating is accompanied by abdominal pain that may be either mild and dull or sharp and intense. Passing gas or having a bowel movement may help to relieve the discomfort.

Most often, bloating results from eating a lot of fatty foods. During the digestive process, fat delays how quickly your stomach empties its contents, which can increase the sensation you may feel of being full. Bloating may also result simply from gulping air while eating too fast.

Sometimes, bloating may be related to an intestinal abnormality, such as celiac disease or lactose intolerance — conditions in which your intestines aren't able to absorb certain food components. Another cause may be fructose intolerance, in which you're unable to properly absorb simple sugars found in fruit and many processed foods.

Bloating may also result from a gastrointestinal infection or from blockage. It may accompany conditions such as irritable bowel syndrome or may be related to stress and anxiety. Bloating may be associated with delayed stomach emptying (gastroparesis), a problem for some people with diabetes.

Intestinal gas

Occasionally, some of the air that you swallow will make it all the way to your colon, where it's expelled through your anus. But most often, intestinal gas (flatus) results from the fermentation of undigested food, such as plant fiber, after it reaches your colon. Gas also forms when your intestines have difficulty breaking down certain components in foods, including the sugars in milk products and fruit.

Constipation can lead to intestinal gas. The longer food waste remains in your colon, the more time it has to ferment. Intestinal gas is composed primarily of odorless substances. The foul smells that may accompany flatulence come from gases containing sulfur that are produced by the decomposing food particles in your colon.

The following practices may help you reduce intestinal gas:

Limit foods that produce gas

Try to identify which foods may be gas-forming for you. Consider that certain foods that produce gas for one person may not produce gas for another person. See the list of foods that commonly produce gas on page 57.

In attempting to relieve your problem, don't eliminate nutritious foods, such as vegetables and fruits, from your diet just because they may cause gas. Generally, you can find ways to reduce gas while maintaining a healthy diet. For example, eat less amounts of a particular food or prepare it in a certain way without the consequences.

Common foods that may promote intestinal gas

Controlling your intake of one of the foods on this list may help you reduce intestinal gas. But remember that different foods affect different people. Do not eliminate these foods from your diet all at one time — you don't want to eliminate the other beneficial nutrients that these foods provide. Instead, try eliminating one food at a time. If your symptoms are reduced, that particular food may be gas-forming for you. Since many factors can cause gas, food thought to be gas-forming should be retested in the future.

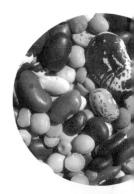

Legumes and certain vegetables

- Baked beans
- Dried beans
- Lima beans
- Broccoli
- Brussels sprouts

- Cabbage
- Cauliflower
- Cucumbers
- Kohlrabi
- Lentils

- Onions
- Dried peas
- Radishes
- Rutabagas
- Sauerkraut

Certain fruits and fruit juices, in excessive amounts

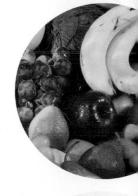

- Apple juice
- Apples
- Bananas

- Prune juice
- Prunes

- Grape juice
- Raisins

Certain dairy products

- Cream
- Ice cream

- Ice milk
- Milk

Many starches, including products made from wheat, potatoes and corn (rice products typically don't produce gas)

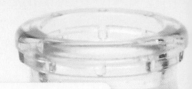

Living with lactose intolerance

You love dairy products, but they don't love you. Shortly after a bowl of ice cream or a serving of cheesy lasagna, you experience cramps, bloating, gas and diarrhea — signs and symptoms that come from a reduced ability to digest milk sugar (lactose). This is a condition called lactose (LAK-tose) intolerance.

To digest lactose, you need the enzyme lactase (LAK-tase). Babies are born with large amounts of lactase. As you grow older, your body often produces less lactase. Adults whose intestines produce very little, if any, lactase have difficulty digesting any foods containing lactose. Between 30 million and 50 million Americans are lactose intolerant.

Tolerance to lactose varies. Most people can handle the amount of lactose in half a cup of milk, and don't have a problem consuming small amounts of dairy products throughout the day. Signs and symptoms occur when they consume several dairy products at one time, or they eat a large portion of a product containing lactose. People with a more severe intolerance aren't able to eat any dairy products without experiencing distressing symptoms.

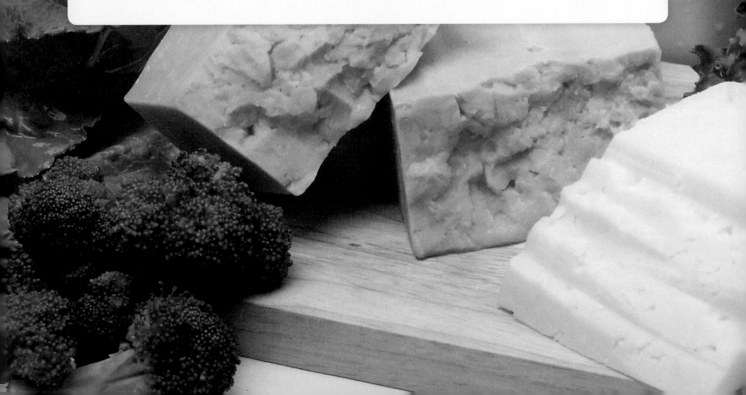

To reduce signs and symptoms of lactose intolerance, avoid these high-lactose foods or eat them in small amounts.

- Cheese spreads
- Chip dip or potato topping
- Cottage cheese
- Dry milk
- Evaporated milk
- **Half-and-half**

- Ice cream or ice milk
- Milk
- Ricotta cheese
- Sour cream
- Sweetened condensed milk
- White sauce

Yogurt is a good food choice because the bacteria in yogurt have already digested much of the lactose in the product. Look for yogurt with active yeast cultures. Other foods that are lower in lactose include aged cheeses, butter, margarine and sherbet. Nondairy creamers are lactose-free.

Tablets or drops sold in stores under brand names such as Lactaid contain the enzyme lactase and can often prevent or relieve symptoms of lactose intolerance. Some milk sold in grocery stores also contains lactase.

Discuss food choices and the elimination of certain foods with your doctor or a registered dietitian. You may try over-the-counter products such as Beano, which reduces gas formation, or one of the many products containing simethicone, intended to relieve gas.

Eating fewer fatty foods, such as fried meats, cream sauces, gravies and rich pastries may help reduce gas. Fatty foods often slow digestion, giving food particles more time to ferment.

The artificial sweeteners sorbitol and mannitol, found in dietetic candies and sugar-free gums, can produce gas. Sweeteners, such as aspartame (Nutra-Sweet, Equal) and saccharin (Sweet'N Low), do not have this side effect.

Add fiber gradually

High-fiber foods are good for digestion and health. But eating too much fiber too quickly can cause gas. Increase the fiber in your diet gradually over a period of several weeks. A dietitian can advise you on which high-fiber foods are less likely to produce gas.

Exercise regularly

Regular exercise reduces intestinal gas by helping to prevent constipation. It may also help get rid of bloating.

Drink plenty of water

Like exercise, water helps to prevent constipation thereby reducing gas.

» *To learn more*

For additional information on conditions that may produce belching, bloating or gas, see these chapters.
Chapter 5: Gastroesophageal reflux disease (GERD)
Chapter 7: Irritable bowel syndrome
Chapter 9: Celiac disease

Indigestion

People frequently visit their doctors for what they call indigestion, a general term that describes discomfort in the upper abdomen. Indigestion is actually a collection of signs and symptoms — uncomfortable fullness, nausea, heartburn and bloating accompanied by belching. Most commonly, though, people associate indigestion with stomach pain (dyspepsia).

Indigestion may be a common complaint for many people but how you experience it may differ from how someone else does. Signs and symptoms may be felt occasionally or as often as every day. Common causes of stomach pain include:

- Peptic ulcers
- Stomach inflammation (gastritis) from medications, alcohol or infection
- Nonulcer dyspepsia, a condition in which people experience symptoms resembling those of an ulcer, although an ulcer doesn't exist

Less commonly, stomach pain or discomfort can be a symptom of other digestive disorders, such as gallbladder inflammation or pancreatic disease.

An occasional episode of dyspepsia generally isn't anything to worry about. It may even be related to hunger pangs. But if you're having persistent, recurrent or severe abdominal pain or discomfort, you should see your doctor.

» **To learn more**

For additional information on conditions that may produce stomach pain or discomfort, see these chapters.
Chapter 6: Ulcers and stomach pain
Chapter 11: Gallstones
Chapter 12: Pancreatitis

Nausea and vomiting

Most people experience an occasional bout of nausea, which is stomach distress accompanied by the urge to vomit. Vomiting is a natural response to invading organisms and irritants in the digestive tract — by forcefully expelling stomach contents.

Often, the culprit is gastroenteritis (gastro-en-tur-I-tis), an inflammation of the lining of the stomach and intestines.

The most common causes are:

- Viral infection
- Bacteria from spoiled food
- High levels of toxins in your blood, including alcohol and drugs
- Increased hormone levels during pregnancy or extended periods of intense stress
- Increased pressure inside your skull due to fluid accumulation or tumor
- Intense headache or inner ear disturbance, including motion sickness

Nausea and vomiting generally aren't signs and symptoms of serious disease unless they persist or they're accompanied by pain. If you can see blood in the vomit or it looks like coffee grounds (partially digested blood), you should see your doctor promptly.

Depending on other signs and symptoms, nausea and vomiting could be caused by a digestive condition that requires medical attention, such as an ulcer, gallstones, pancreatitis, liver disease or intestinal obstruction.

Self-care

For infrequent nausea and vomiting due to a virus or bacterium, the following may help limit your discomfort and prevent dehydration:

- Stop eating and drinking for several hours until your stomach has had a chance to settle.
- Avoid food odors. Eat cold foods or those that don't require cooking.
- When you begin to feel better, suck on ice chips or take small sips of water, weak tea, clear soft drinks, noncaffeinated sports drinks or broth. Sip beverages often to prevent dehydration.
- Gradually add easily digested foods, such as gelatin, crackers and dry toast. Once you can tolerate these, try mild-flavored, nonfatty foods such as cereal, rice and fruits.

- For several days, avoid fatty or spicy foods, caffeine, alcohol, and aspirin or other nonsteroidal anti-inflammatory drugs (NSAIDs).

» *To learn more*

For additional information on conditions that may produce nausea and vomiting, see these chapters.
Chapter 6: Ulcers and stomach pain
Chapter 11: Gallstones
Chapter 12: Pancreatitis
Chapter 13: Liver disease

Abdominal pain

Abdominal pain can occur on its own, or it may accompany other digestive signs and symptoms. Occasional episodes of pain often stem from overeating or eating too much of the wrong foods, such as fatty foods, gas-producing foods or, for people with lactose intolerance, dairy products. Usually the pain goes away within a few hours. In case of a viral or bacterial infection, discomfort may linger for one or two days.

Abdominal pain that's recurrent, persistent, severe or accompanied by other signs and symptoms may signal a potentially serious condition. Where the pain is located in your abdomen may help your doctor narrow the list of possible causes. However, sometimes the location can be misleading.

Navel area

Pain near your navel often is related to a disorder of the small intestine or an inflammation of your appendix (appendicitis). The appendix is a worm-shaped pouch that projects out from your colon. It can become clogged with food waste that causes it to inflame, swell and fill with pus. Without treatment, an infected appendix can burst and cause a serious infection (peritonitis).

In addition to pain around your navel, which can spread to your lower right abdomen, other signs and symptoms of appendicitis may include nausea, vomiting, loss of appetite, low-grade fever, and the urge to pass gas or have a bowel movement.

Above the navel

The epigastric area is located in the center of your abdomen and directly above the naval. This is where you should expect to feel pain associated with stomach disorders. Persistent pain in this area also may signal a problem with your upper small intestine (duodenum), pancreas or gallbladder.

Below the navel

Pain that's located below the navel, and spreading out to either side, may signify a disorder of the colon, or large intestine. Other common causes of pain in this area may be the result of a urinary tract infection, pelvic inflammatory disease or ovarian conditions in women.

Upper left abdomen

It's uncommon to experience pain in the upper left area of the abdomen. When you do, it may suggest a problem in the colon, stomach or pancreas.

Upper right abdomen

Intense pain in the upper right area of the abdomen is often related to an inflammation of the gallbladder (gallbladder attack). The pain may spread to the center of your abdomen and penetrate to your back. Occasionally, an inflammation in your pancreas or duodenum and even some liver disorders can produce intense pain in this area.

Lower left abdomen

Pain in the lower left area of the abdomen most often suggests a problem in your descending sigmoid colon (the section just above the rectum). Possible disorders include an infection in the colon (diverticulitis), colon cancer or inflammation of the colon (Crohn's disease or ulcerative colitis).

Lower right abdomen

Pain in the lower right area of the abdomen may indicate an inflammation of the colon or the end of the small intestine (terminal ileum). It may also indicate certain diseases of the colon, such as Crohn's disease or colon cancer. Sometimes, appendicitis may be a possible cause of pain in this area.

Migrating pain

An unusual characteristic of abdominal pain is its ability to travel along deep nerve pathways and emerge at locations that are some distance away from the true source of the problem. For example, pain from gallbladder inflammation may spread to your chest and up to your right shoulder. Pain from a pancreatic disorder may radiate up between your shoulder blades. Your doctor calls this referred pain.

Because of the number of vital organs in your abdomen, and the complex signals they send, it's a good idea to consult your doctor if you experience any of the following:

- Severe, recurrent or persistent pain
- Pain that seems to worsen
- Pain accompanied by fever, bleeding or vomiting

Consider that abdominal pain that persists or recurs — regardless of its location — can sometimes be due to cancer, especially in older adults.

There are many treatment options to manage pain. Your best approach is to have a thorough medical evaluation of the kind of pain you're experiencing and the effect it's having on you.

In the meantime, find ways to ease pain. For instance, eat smaller meals if your pain is accompanied by indigestion. Avoid taking over-the-counter pain relievers such as aspirin or ibuprofen (Advil, Motrin, others) because these can cause stomach problems that may worsen abdominal pain.

» *To learn more*

For additional information on conditions that may produce abdominal pain, see these chapters.

Diarrhea and constipation

These are common signs and symptoms that virtually everyone will experience at one time or another in his or her life. Typically, diarrhea or constipation lasts for a short period and then disappears. But sometimes, it can be persistent. Persistent signs and symptoms generally signal a digestive disorder.

Diarrhea

Diarrhea is a change toward a more liquid consistency of your stool, an increased frequency in passing stool, an increase in the amount of stool you pass — and often some combination of all three developments during a given period of time. Diarrhea often results when the lining of your small intestine becomes inflamed, which hampers the ability of your intestinal tract to absorb nutrients and fluids.

Ordinarily after a meal, nutrients from the food and liquid you've consumed are processed and absorbed in your small intestine. Your colon absorbs the remaining liquid from digested food, and waste forms into semisolid stools. Diarrhea occurs when this process is disrupted.

There are various agents that can interrupt the digestive process, impeding the absorption of nutrients and fluids:

Viral infection
This is the most common cause of diarrhea. An invading virus damages the mucous membrane that lines your small intestine, disrupting fluid and nutrient absorption. Typically, after one to three days, symptoms begin to improve and the diarrhea gradually disappears.

Bacterial infection
Bacteria in contaminated food or water form a toxin that causes the intestines to secrete salt and water. This overwhelms the capacity of your small intestine and colon to absorb fluid. As with a viral infection, the diarrhea that results usually lasts one to three days.

Other infectious agents
Though much less common, diarrhea may result from a parasite. Once the parasite is eliminated, the diarrhea usually disappears.

Medications
Diarrhea may also result from medications such as certain antacids that contain magnesium hydroxide or from certain antibiotics. Once the medication is discontinued, the diarrhea usually goes away.

Intestinal disorders

Diarrhea that persists or recurs frequently is usually related to some form of intestinal disorder. Possible causes include irritable bowel syndrome, an inflammatory disease such as ulcerative colitis or Crohn's disease, or a malabsorption condition such as lactose intolerance or celiac disease. Sometimes diarrhea is associated with a tumor.

Excessive caffeine or alcohol

Caffeinated and alcoholic beverages can stimulate the passage of stool. If you drink them in excess, they may cause food waste to move through your small intestine and colon too quickly.

Self-care

Diarrhea ordinarily clears up on its own, without the need for antibiotics or other medications. There are some over-the-counter products, such as Imodium, Pepto-Bismol and Kaopectate, that may slow diarrhea, but these products won't always speed your recovery. Severe diarrhea, persistent or recurrent abdominal pain, or bleeding should prompt a visit to your doctor.

Dehydration can often become a major concern because diarrhea greatly increases the amount of fluid you would typically lose in a day. Take these measures to prevent dehydration and relieve symptoms as you recover.

Drink plenty of fluids

Drink at least eight to 10 glasses of clear liquid daily. This includes water, weak tea, diluted juices, or beverages containing electrolytes, such as Gatorade or Powerade.

Gradually add solid foods

Start your recovery with easily digestible food, such as crackers, toast, rice, cereal and chicken.

Avoid certain foods and beverages

Wait a few days before consuming dairy products, fatty foods, spicy foods, or beverages containing caffeine or alcohol. They can prolong diarrhea.

Don't take certain antacids

Magnesium hydroxide can cause diarrhea, so avoid any products that contain this substance.

Reduce stress

For some forms of chronic diarrhea, therapies such as acupuncture, acupressure or massage may reduce symptoms by relieving stress and stimulating your body's natural defense systems. However, none of these therapies has been scientifically proved.

What over-the-counter products help constipation?

Lifestyle changes are the best and safest way to manage constipation. If they don't help, or their benefits seem limited, you might try a natural fiber supplement, such as psyllium (Metamucil) or methylcellulose (Citrucel). These products often relieve constipation within weeks. Fiber supplements are generally safe, but because they're so absorbent, take them with plenty of water. If you don't drink enough water, the supplements can become constipating — the opposite result of what you want. Start with a small amount of the supplement and increase that amount slowly every one to two weeks.

Laxatives also relieve constipation, but talk to your doctor before taking any laxative. If used for more than a few days, laxatives can be harmful. Stool softeners, such as Colace, Correctol, Stool Softener and Surfak, are the most gentle products. Saline (osmotic) laxatives, such as Phillips' Milk of Magnesia and Miralax, also are relatively safe. Stimulant laxatives, including Dulcolax, Ex-Lax and Senokot, are the most powerful products.

Constipation

One of your colon's main responsibilities is to absorb water from food residue as it moves through. For as long as food residue remains in your colon, it loses its water content. If it stays for a long time, the waste becomes very dry and difficult to pass as stool.

How long between bowel movements is too long? It varies. Some people have two or three bowel movements each day. Others have bowel movements only three or four times a week. However, if you have bowel movements just once or twice a week, or you have to strain to pass stool, chances are that you're constipated.

Constipation can occur for many reasons, and it tends to be more common with age. As you get older, the muscles in your digestive tract become less active, which means food is not moved as easily as before. Your lifestyle also may change. Factors that increase your risk of constipation include not drinking enough liquids, eating too little fiber and not getting enough exercise.

In addition, certain medications can slow digestion, producing constipation. They include narcotics and antacids containing aluminum. Some people with irritable bowel syndrome experience alternating episodes of diarrhea and constipation.

Generally, constipation is a temporary condition that can be easily corrected. However, there are times when constipation may point to a more serious problem.

See your doctor if you experience:

- Recent, unexplained onset of constipation
- Recent, unexplained change in bowel patterns or habits
- Constipation that lasts longer than seven days, despite changes in diet or exercise
- Blood in stool or intense abdominal pain

Self-care

These tips often can help relieve or prevent constipation.

Drink plenty of fluids
Drink at least eight to 10 glasses of clear liquid daily. Liquid helps keep your stool soft. Water is preferable.

Eat high-fiber foods
Fiber helps bulk up and soften stool so that it passes smoothly through your digestive tract.

For adults age 50 and younger, the daily dietary recommendations are 38 grams (g) of fiber for men and 25 g for women. For adults older than 50, the recommendations are 30 g for men and 21 g for women.

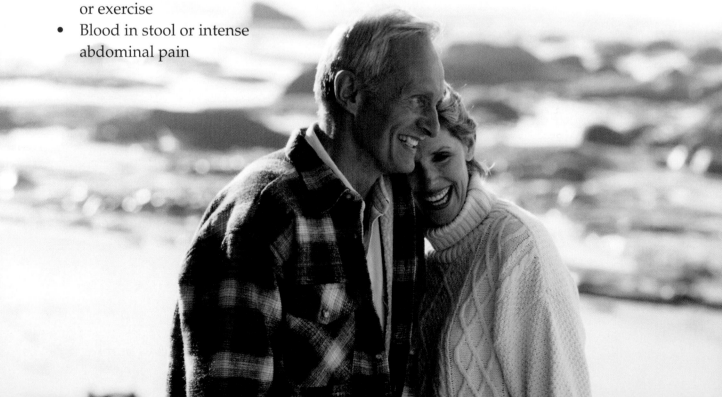

Whole grains, fruits and vegetables are your best fiber sources (see "Where to find fiber" on pages 33-34).

To avoid abdominal gas, cramping and bloating that can occur from adding too much fiber to your diet too quickly, it's best to gradually increase the total amount of fiber you eat over a period of several weeks.

Enjoy regular meals

Eating on a regular schedule promotes normal bowel function, especially when you eat breakfast early in the day.

Exercise regularly

Exercise stimulates your gastrointestinal muscles, hastening the passage of food through your digestive tract. Try to exercise for 30 to 60 minutes on most, if not all, days of the week.

Heed nature's call

When you feel the urge, the longer you delay going to the bathroom, the more water that's absorbed from food waste and the harder your stool becomes. Don't linger on the toilet, but relax and give yourself enough time to complete your bowel movement.

Reduce stress

Stress can slow digestion. For some forms of chronic constipation, practices such as yoga, massage, acupressure or aromatherapy may reduce symptoms by relieving stress and promoting relaxation. However, none of these therapies has been scientifically proved.

» *To learn more*

For additional information on conditions that may produce diarrhea or constipation, see these chapters.

Chapter 7: Irritable bowel syndrome
Chapter 8: Crohn's disease and ulcerative colitis
Chapter 9: Celiac disease
Chapter 10: Diverticular disease
Chapter 12: Pancreatitis
Chapter 14: Cancer

Bleeding

You can easily become alarmed if you notice traces of blood coming from either your mouth or your anus — the two endpoints of your digestive tract. Sometimes the bleeding may be a minor problem, such as gum disease or hemorrhoids. At other times, the bleeding is warning of a more serious condition, such as an ulcer or cancer. The safest course of action is to see your doctor as soon as possible.

Blood in saliva or vomit

Blood may come from many sources, including injury to the mouth, gums or nose. If you cough up blood, the source is usually the lungs or windpipe. Digestive conditions that may cause blood to exit from your mouth in saliva or vomit include the following:

- Peptic ulcer
- Tear in the lining of your esophagus
- Inflamed tissue in your esophagus, stomach or small intestine
- Cancer of the esophagus or stomach

The blood is usually bright red. Occasionally, it may appear black or dark brown and resemble coffee grounds, which means it has been partly digested in your stomach or duodenum. This often indicates a serious problem that should be investigated.

Call for emergency assistance if you vomit blood. While waiting for help, lie down with legs elevated, if possible. Don't attempt to eat or drink anything.

Rectal bleeding

Bleeding from the rectum and anus can be the result of many problems. It may show up as blood in your stool, on used toilet paper or in the toilet bowel. Often the underlying cause of rectal bleeding can be treated. See your doctor to determine what's causing your symptoms.

An anal tear (fissure) and hemorrhoids are the most frequent causes of rectal bleeding (see "Harmless but troublesome hemorrhoids" on pages 71-72). The blood is usually bright red.

Other causes of rectal bleeding include inflammation of the colon caused by ulcerative colitis or Crohn's disease. Rectal bleeding can also be a warning of noncancerous growths (polyps) or cancer in the colon.

Sometimes, the blood is darker in color and mixed in with stool, producing black, maroon or mahogany-colored stools. Black stools may indicate bleeding from the upper intestine.

» *To learn more*

For additional information on conditions that may produce bleeding, see these chapters.
Chapter 6: Ulcers and stomach pain
Chapter 8: Crohn's disease and ulcerative colitis
Chapter 14: Cancer

Harmless but troublesome hemorrhoids

Sometimes, you may not even know they're there. Other times, bleeding, itching or burning pain in the rectal area lets you know that you have hemorrhoids.

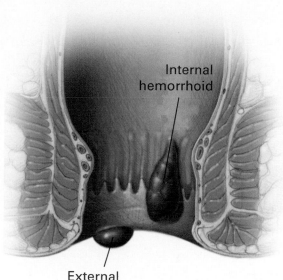

Internal hemorrhoid

External hemorrhoid

Hemorrhoids are swollen, blood-engorged veins in your anus and lower rectum. The swelling comes from pressure put on the veins, causing them to stretch and form tiny sacs. Bleeding may occur because the veins are easily ruptured. Hemorrhoids are common. By age 50, about half of adults have had to deal with them.

Constipation and diarrhea are common causes of hemorrhoids. Frequent straining to pass small, hard stools increases pressure on the veins. So does the abrupt expulsion of loose stools. Other causes of hemorrhoids include lifting heavy objects, sitting or standing for long periods, obesity and pregnancy.

Hemorrhoids can occur internally near the beginning of the anal canal or externally, where they protrude outside the anus. Both types are common and both may bleed. Avoid dry, rough toilet paper because it can irritate hemorrhoids. After a bowel movement, clean your anus carefully with a warm washcloth or a medicated wipe. If you do detect rectal bleeding, don't assume it's from hemorrhoids — see your doctor.

continued >

Often, treatment for hemorrhoids involves steps that you can take on your own. You can treat most hemorrhoids by increasing the fiber and water in your diet, to soften your stools. Soaking in a warm bath for 10 to 15 minutes at least two to three times a day may relieve swelling and pain. Over-the-counter hemorrhoid creams, ointments or pads containing the astringent witch hazel, or a topical anesthetic agent also can relieve swelling and pain.

Sometimes, minimally invasive procedures or surgery is necessary to take care of troublesome hemorrhoids. One such procedure is rubber band ligation. Your doctor places one or two tiny rubber bands around the base of an internal hemorrhoid to cut off its circulation. The hemorrhoid withers and falls off within a few days. With a procedure known as sclerotherapy, a chemical solution is injected around the blood vessel to shrink the hemorrhoid. Surgery to remove a severe hemorrhoid is known as hemorrhoidectomy.

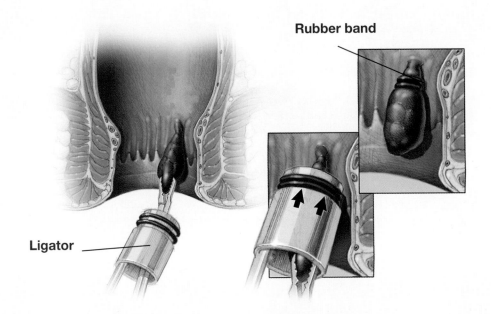

Rubber band

Ligator

To remove an internal hemorrhoid with a rubber band, a doctor first attaches a special instrument (ligator) to the hemorrhoid and stretches it downward (left). A rubber band is then placed around the hemorrhoid to cut off its blood supply (right).

Weight loss

For people who spend years struggling to shed a few pounds, unintentional weight loss might seem like a gift. However, losing a significant amount of weight without really trying can indicate a serious medical disorder, and should be discussed with your doctor.

Everyone's weight tends to fluctuate from day to day and week to week. You should expect a little variation whenever you step on a bathroom scale to weigh yourself.

But what if you notice you're losing weight even though your daily routine is unchanged, you're eating and exercising just as you always have and you're not on a diet? Involuntary weight loss is defined as a loss of more than 5 percent of your body weight over a six-month span. That means, if you typically weigh around 160 pounds, a 5 percent loss would be about 8 pounds.

Even if you're unsure of what your original weight was, you can look for other clues that may indicate you're losing weight. For example, you may notice that your clothes fit more loosely, or that you may be fastening your belt at a tighter notch.

The list of potential causes for involuntary weight loss is extensive. The first thing many people worry about is cancer, but a majority won't have it. Digestive conditions that may lead to involuntary weight loss include:

- Difficulty swallowing
- Malabsorption disorders
- Pancreas or liver disease
- Cancer

If you're losing weight and you're not sure why, see your doctor. In preparing for the visit, list any other signs and symptoms you may be experiencing. The management of involuntary weight loss involves determining what's producing the loss. Once a cause has been identified, your doctor will be better able to treat the problem. If you and your doctor think that the weight loss is significant, you may need to undergo some diagnostic testing.

» *To learn more*

For additional information on conditions that may produce weight loss, see these chapters.

Chapter 4

Diagnostic tests

For most people, an occasional bout of heartburn or diarrhea is not much cause for alarm. It's when digestive symptoms persist or worsen that people usually turn to their doctors. Giving you a physical examination and asking a series of questions about your signs and symptoms and daily routine may be all that your doctor needs to diagnose what's wrong.

Sometimes, before a diagnosis can be made, your doctor may need to perform one or more specialized tests. These tests are especially helpful when a number of possible causes could be producing your symptoms — the results may be able to point to or eliminate one or more of the possibilities. Testing may also be done later to help confirm the initial diagnosis.

There are many different kinds of diagnostic tests for digestive conditions. Which tests are used will depend, in part, on what your signs and symptoms are, as well as on their location, severity and frequency. Other factors in the selection may include your age, general health and family medical history. All of this may be determined during the initial interview with your doctor.

The diagnostic tests described in this chapter are the most common ones used for digestive conditions. Some of these tests generate detailed pictures of inside your body, allowing the doctor to see the size and structure of your internal organs and, possibly, the presence of tumors, growths (polyps), narrowed areas (strictures) and other abnormalities. Other tests track how different parts of your digestive system are performing, for example, by measuring the strength of muscle contractions in your esophagus or determining how quickly food passes through your intestinal tract.

Tracking may be accomplished with a laboratory analysis of samples such as blood or urine that's collected from your body, or by studying special images taken of your digestive system at work. Types of imaging include radiologic and endoscopic.

Radiologic imaging is produced when a form of energy — such as X-rays, sound waves, magnetic fields or radioactive particles — is transmitted through your body. When this energy encounters body tissues of different densities, special devices capture changes in the energy pattern and convert this information into a picture. Radiologic tests include X-ray, ultrasound, computerized tomography (CT), and magnetic resonance imaging (MRI).

Endoscopic imaging involves threading a thin, flexible tube into your body that's equipped with a viewing lens or video camera, permitting the doctor to see directly inside. The doctor or a technician controls the movement and position of the tube, or "scope," to display a real-time image on an external monitor. Endoscopic tests include enteroscopy (into the small intestine) and colonoscopy or sigmoidoscopy (into the colon).

Diagnostic tests such as these can provide valuable information about the different organs or processes in your digestive system but still may not be able to identify the exact cause of your problem. For example, a cause for abdominal pain or nausea can often be difficult to pinpoint. Sometimes, your diagnosis is reached through a process of elimination, guided by the results of multiple tests.

The following sections begin with the tests that your doctor often starts with in the diagnostic process, and then move on to more specialized or less commonly required tests.

Blood tests

Blood tests often are a first step in the diagnostic process because they're relatively simple to perform and can provide a general idea of what's going on inside your body. They require little preparation. Using a syringe, the doctor draws a sample of blood, usually from a vein in your arm.

Depending on your signs and symptoms, one or more of following blood tests may be necessary.

Complete blood count (CBC)

This test measures several properties of blood, including levels of red cells and white cells. Fewer red blood cells (anemia), and lower hemoglobin found within the red cells, may be associated with gastrointestinal bleeding. An elevated level of white blood cells may indicate infection or inflammation.

Liver tests

These tests measure levels of certain enzymes and proteins in your blood. If your liver is not functioning properly, the levels often are abnormal. For more on liver disease, see Chapter 13.

Measurements of albumin, vitamins D, A and B-12, and folate

Abnormal levels of these substances in your blood suggest that your intestines may not be absorbing certain nutrients from food properly — typically, a malabsorption problem.

Electrolyte measurements

Severe vomiting or diarrhea can cause abnormal blood levels of the electrolytes sodium and potassium. A very low level of potassium can put you at risk of heart problems.

Urine and stool tests

A urine test can help identify abnormal levels of hormones, proteins, minerals or salts in your urine, or the presence of substances not normally found in urine such as blood. This knowledge can guide diagnosis and medical care.

Your doctor may request a stool sample to check for parasites or bacteria (or their associated toxins), which may be the cause of severe diarrhea. Stool tests can also identify increased levels of fat in your stool, suggesting a malabsorption problem.

Another common stool test is a fecal occult blood test. This test checks for hidden (occult) blood in your stool, which may be linked to cancer or other diseases that may cause intestinal bleeding, such as ulcers or inflammatory bowel disease.

A fecal occult blood test may become a routine part of colorectal cancer screening for people age 50 or older. However, not all cancer lesions or precancerous polyps bleed and those that do often bleed intermittently. Therefore, it's possible to get a negative test result even though cancer is present.

Stool DNA test

The stool DNA test is a new screening approach for the detection of colorectal cancer. Here's how the test is designed to work. The lining of your colon continually sheds cells, which leave the body through your stool. Cells from the surface of precancerous polyps and cancerous tumors show recognizable DNA changes (DNA markers). A stool DNA test identifies several of these markers, which indicate the presence of the precancerous polyps or colon cancer to your doctor. One test is currently available but has not been certified by the Food and Drug Administration. Other tests are being developed and still require full clinical validation. Use of the stool DNA test has been endorsed by various institutions, including the American Cancer Society and the American College of Radiology.

Certain foods, such as broccoli, cauliflower and undercooked red meat, contain chemicals that can produce a false reading, suggesting the presence of blood in stool when there isn't any. Just the opposite, vitamin C supplements can mask a positive reaction.

A similar test for blood in stool, called the HemoQuant test, was developed at Mayo Clinic. It's less likely to give false readings but it's more expensive and administering the test is more involved.

Most doctors, including physicians at Mayo Clinic, recommend other screening methods for colorectal cancer instead of, or in addition to, fecal occult blood tests. These include sigmoidoscopy, colonoscopy, barium enema and CT colonography. These tests are described later in this chapter.

X-rays

X-ray imaging tests are other early options in the diagnosis of digestive problems because, like blood tests, they're relatively simple to perform. They involve exposing a part of your body to a small dose of electromagnetic radiation, which passes through bones, organs and soft tissue. Special film positioned on the other side of your body collects the signals, generating a 2-D image of your internal structures. There are different kinds of X-rays, and the kind of test you undergo will depend on the location of your symptoms.

Upper gastrointestinal X-ray

This test uses X-ray images to look for problems in your esophagus, stomach and upper portion of the small intestine (duodenum). Fasting before the procedure helps clear food and eliminate liquid from your stomach, making it easier to detect abnormalities.

At the beginning of the procedure, you swallow a thick, white liquid containing barium, a soft, metallic alkaline chemical. The barium temporarily coats the lining of your digestive tract and makes the lining show up more clearly on X-ray films. You may also be asked to swallow gas-producing liquid or pills, such as sodium bicarbonate. This stretches your stomach, separating its folds and providing a better view of the inner lining.

A radiologist will position an X-ray machine above you, if you're lying down, or in front of you, if you're standing. Exposing your body to a small dose of radiation allows the radiologist to follow the progress of the barium through your upper gastrointestinal

tract on a video monitor and detect problems in how your digestive system works. For instance, X-rays can help show if the muscles that control swallowing are functioning properly as they contract and relax. X-ray images can also detect a narrowing (stricture) of your esophagus, as well as ulcers, tumors and other abnormalities in your stomach and duodenum.

The upper gastrointestinal (GI) X-ray procedure itself may take 20 to 45 minutes, depending on what the radiologist sees. The barium eventually passes through your entire digestive tract, producing white stools for a few days afterward. Constipation is sometimes a side effect, which may be prevented by drinking plenty of fluids. Your doctor may recommend that you use a laxative, enema or combination of the two to help eliminate the barium.

Small intestine (small bowel) X-ray

If your doctor suspects a problem in your small intestine, such as an obstruction, the procedure may be expanded to include your entire small intestine — the jejunum and ileum as well as the duodenum. X-ray images are generally taken at 15- to 30-minute intervals as the barium moves through each section. It can take up to four hours for the barium to reach the end of the small intestine (terminal ileum). Once the barium reaches your colon, the test is finished. You may use a laxative or enema to help clear the barium.

Colon X-ray (barium enema)

Barium enema is a name commonly used for a X-ray of the colon, or large intestine. This test allows your doctor to examine your entire colon, looking for ulcers, strictures, polyps, small pouches in the lining (diverticula), tumors and other abnormalities.

Your colon needs to be empty for this procedure, so for one to two days beforehand you may need to restrict your diet to clear liquids, such as broth, gelatin, coffee, tea and soft drinks. You will also be given laxatives, and perhaps enemas, before the test to help empty your colon.

During the procedure you lie on an examination table beneath an X-ray machine. The radiologist places a slender, lubricated tube into your rectum. This tube is connected to a bag of barium that coats the walls of your colon so that its lining will show up more clearly on the X-ray. As the barium drains into your colon from the bag above you,

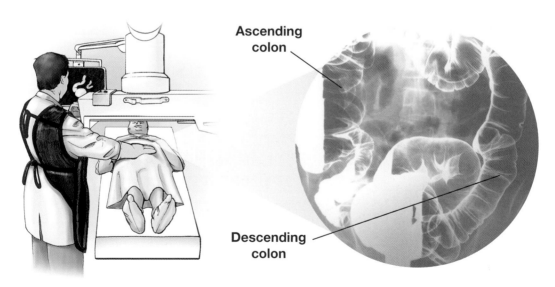

Ascending colon

Descending colon

A colon X-ray exam begins when a tube inserted into your rectum releases barium to highlight your colon's inner lining. Air may be pumped through the tube to inflate the colon and improve visibility. The radiologist views your colon on an external monitor to select the best images.

you'll feel the urge for a bowel movement. A small balloon attached to the tube, located in your lower colon, helps keep the barium from leaking back out.

The radiologist will study your colon's shape and condition on a monitor attached to the X-ray machine. As barium fills your colon, you will be asked to turn and hold several positions to provide different views of your colon. At times, the radiologist may press firmly on your abdomen and pelvis to manipulate your colon for better viewing.

The radiologist also may inject air through the tubing to expand your colon and improve the image. This form of testing is called a double- or air-contrast barium enema.

After the exam, which generally takes about 20 to 40 minutes, the radiologist will lower the barium bag, allowing much of the barium to drain out of your colon. This will make you feel more comfortable.

For a few days afterward, you'll probably have white or gray stools while the rest of the barium leaves your system. Drink plenty of liquids during this time to prevent constipation. Your doctor may suggest that you use enemas or a laxative to help clear out the barium.

Computerized tomography

Computerized tomography (CT) combines X-rays with computer technology to produce 3-D images of your internal organs and other tissues. The procedure detects many different levels of tissue density — in contrast to standard X-rays that detect only a few levels of density — providing greater detail and clarity on the images.

CT is an effective imaging procedure for diagnosing tumors, accumulations of blood or other fluids, or infections (abscesses) deep inside your body, as well as intestinal hernias, obstructions and perforations.

For the procedure, you lie on an examination table that slides into a doughnut-shaped X-ray scanner. The scanner will rotate around you, taking a sequence of very narrow scans from many different angles. A detector rotates opposite the scanner, on the other side of your body, collecting the signals. A computer collects and combines the signals into a 3-D image of your internal structures that the radiologist can examine from any angle, or dissect into cross-sectional layers. The radiologist is able to view each layer separately.

CT scans of your abdomen and pelvis can help identify abnormalities in your pancreas, spleen, liver and kidneys, and sometimes your stomach, intestines, gallbladder, bile ducts and other pelvic organs.

An abdominal CT scan is painless. You may need to fast before the scan, which helps clear your gastrointestinal tract, making it easier to see the digestive organs and the presence of any abnormalities. The doctor may also ask you to take a laxative or have an enema.

The most uncomfortable part of the abdominal CT procedure may be drinking (or receiving by injection) a liquid containing iodine — the taste of which may be unpleasant. The liquid serves as a contrast agent during the procedure, making your organs and tissues show up more clearly on the scan.

Because some people are allergic to iodine, before the test begins you'll be asked if you've ever had an allergic reaction to iodine or similar contrast agents used in radiologic tests.

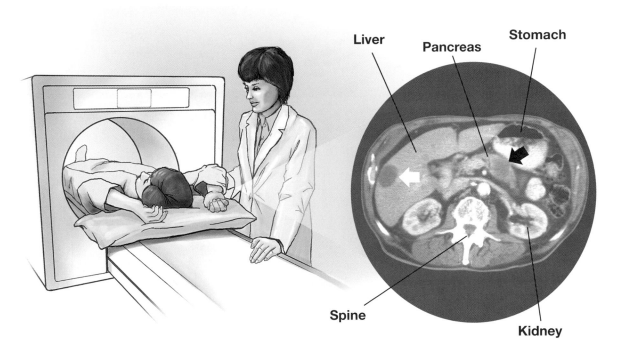

During computerized tomography (CT), a X-ray scanner rotates around you, taking scans from different angles as your examination table slides through the ring. The example at right of a CT cross-sectional scan reveals a tumor on the pancreas (black arrow) which has spread to the liver (white arrow).

Ultrasound

Ultrasound, also called sonography, uses the reflection of high-frequency sound waves to produce pictures of your internal organs — similar in principle to the underwater sonar technology that's used onboard ships.

While you lie on an examination table, a wand-like device (transducer) is pressed against your abdomen. The transducer transmits inaudible sound waves into your body that bounce off internal structures with different tissue densities. The reflected waves are captured by the transducer. A computer translates this data into a moving, 2-D image that's displayed on an external monitor. The exam is painless and usually takes less than 30 minutes.

Ultrasound is often used to examine abdominal organs such as your liver, pancreas, gallbladder, pelvic organs, aorta and kidneys. It's especially useful in detecting gallstones and excess fluid (ascites) within the abdominal cavity.

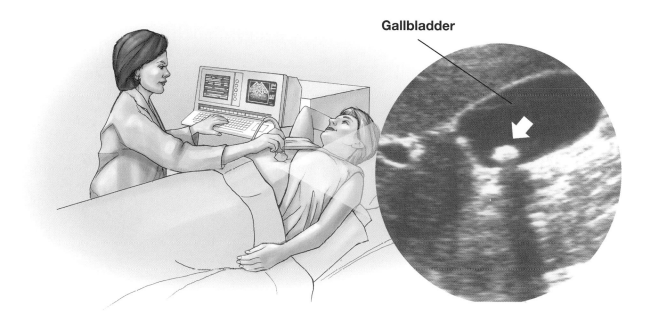

Gallbladder

During ultrasound, reflected sound waves emitted from the hand-held transducer are collected and turned into a moving, 2-D picture on an external monitor. The scan at right reveals a large gallstone in the gallbladder (white arrow).

Using special techniques, ultrasound can also determine the flow of blood in arteries and veins, helping to identify blockage or obstruction.

Endoscopy

One of the most effective ways for your doctor to diagnose digestive problems is to look directly inside your digestive tract. To do this, a thin, flexible tube equipped with a fiber-optic light and tiny electronic camera is inserted into your body.

The tube can be inserted via one of two primary routes. The first route is down through your mouth and then through your esophagus, stomach and upper small intestine (duodenum). The alternate route is up through your anus and then through your rectum and all or part of your colon, even into terminal ileum of the small intestine.

An endoscope (EN-do-skope) is the instrument that your doctor uses to examine the gastrointestinal tract. When used to examine the lower gastrointestinal tract, the endoscope is typically referred to as a colonoscope (ko-LON-o-skope) or, in a shorter version, a sigmoidoscope (sig-MOI-do-skope).

Upper endoscopy

This procedure (esophagogastroduodenoscopy, or EGD) allows your doctor look directly inside your esophagus, stomach and duodenum. The images from this test help determine what might be causing signs and symptoms of the upper gastrointestinal tract such as difficulty swallowing, heartburn, nausea, vomiting, chest pain, bleeding or upper abdominal pain.

During an EGD, the doctor will look for inflamed tissue, ulcers and abnormal growths. Small instruments may be inserted through the endoscope to perform a variety of delicate procedures:

- Take tissue samples (biopsies)
- Remove foreign objects or noncancerous growths (polyps)
- Stretch (dilate) your esophagus if it's narrowed by scar tissue
- Identify and treat bleeding lesions

Your stomach needs to be empty for the test, so you can't eat or drink anything for at least four to six hours before the examination. Right before the procedure, you may receive medication through a vein that sedates you. You may also receive an anesthetic spray to numb your throat and help prevent you from gagging.

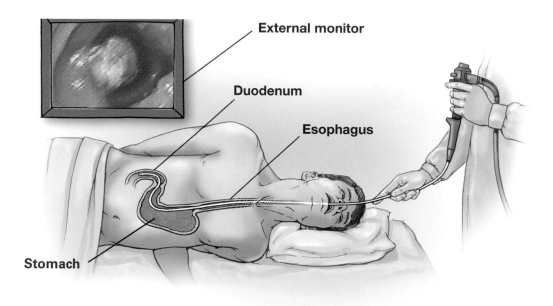

External monitor

Duodenum

Esophagus

Stomach

An endoscope provides a real-time image of your upper gastrointestinal tract, including your esophagus, stomach and duodenum. Images from inside the digestive tract appear on an external monitor.

After placing the endoscope in your mouth, your doctor will ask you to swallow to help pass the tube from your throat into your esophagus. The tube doesn't interfere with your breathing, but you may feel mild pressure or fullness as it moves slowly through your digestive tract. En route, the small camera transmits pictures, allowing your doctor to carefully examine the lining of your esophagus, stomach and upper small intestine for abnormalities.

Abnormalities that don't show up as well on an X-ray image are now more visible, such as inflamed esophageal tissue from stomach reflux and abnormally dilated blood vessels (varices) in

your esophagus. The doctor can also locate small ulcers and tumors in your stomach and duodenum.

For a better view of the stomach lining, air may be blown in to inflate your stomach and stretch out its natural folds. The air may cause you to belch or pass gas afterward.

EGD generally takes about 15 minutes, but you'll need an hour or more to recover from the sedative. You'll also need someone to drive you home, since the effects of the sedative may linger for 24 hours. The endoscope can sometimes cause your throat to feel mildly sore or irritated for a day or two.

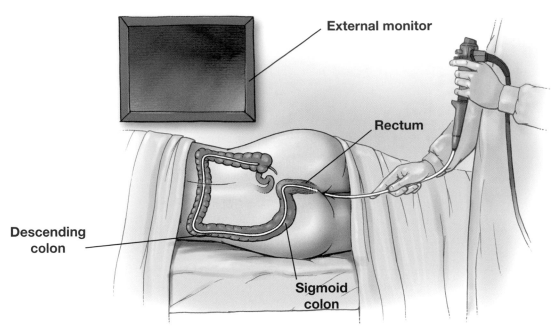

External monitor

Rectum

Descending colon

Sigmoid colon

During colonoscopy a flexible endoscope is inserted into your rectum and threaded through the length of your colon. Images of the lower gastrointestinal tract appear on an external monitor.

Colonoscopy

A similar procedure to the upper endoscopy, a colonoscopy allows your doctor to visually examine your lower digestive tract. While studying the visuals as the scope moves through your colon, the doctor can:

- Inspect for abnormalities, such as bleeding, blood vessels, ulcers, inflammation, polyps, tumors, pouches (diverticula) and narrowed areas
- Take biopsy samples
- Remove polyps
- Treat bleeding lesions
- Stretch (dilate) narrowed areas

Your colon needs to be empty for this procedure. Just as with a colon X-ray, you'll be placed on a clear-liquid diet for one to two days beforehand. You will also be given laxatives and perhaps an enema. Just before the exam, you'll likely receive a sedative through a vein to help you relax. You may also be given a pain reliever.

During the exam, you lie on your left side. The colonoscope has a channel that allows your doctor to pump air into your colon. This inflates the colon for a better view of the interior walls.

Colonoscopy on average takes about 30 minutes, but may take longer depend-

Virtual colonoscopy

Computerized tomography (CT) colonography, also known as virtual colonoscopy, is an imaging technique that combines and digitally manipulates CT images of your abdominal organs to produce a detailed view of the inside of the colon and rectum. Unlike conventional colonoscopy, virtual colonoscopy does not require sedation or the insertion of an endoscope into the colon. Typically, it's used for screening people who are at average risk of colorectal cancer and for those unable to tolerate a traditional colonoscopy.

Before the scan, you're given laxatives to clear your colon of stool. To begin the exam, your colon is filled with air or carbon dioxide by inserting a small catheter inside the rectum. Images are then made of the entire colon and rectum with a CT scanner.

Virtual colonoscopy is usually faster than traditional colonoscopy. A scan of your entire colon generally takes about 10 minutes. At times you may be asked to hold your breath to limit your abdominal movement and avoid distorting the images. In some cases, a contrast dye is given intravenously to highlight polyps in the colon.

Recent studies comparing the results of virtual colonoscopy with traditional colonoscopy have found that the new procedure is often as sensitive in detecting polyps over one quarter inch diameter as traditional colonoscopy. However, if suspect areas are found, you'll need traditional colonoscopy to get a better view of the area, to perform biopsies and to remove the polyps. Researchers are studying whether virtual colonoscopy can be done successfully without prior bowel preparation.

Virtual colonoscopy is not the test of choice for people who are at high risk of precancerous polyps because it's highly likely that the traditional procedure will be required anyway.

ing on whether additional procedures, such as polyp removal, are necessary. You'll feel some cramping or pressure during the exam, which should end when the scope is removed.

Once the exam is over, it takes an hour or more to recover from the sedative. You'll also need someone to drive you home because it takes up to a day for the full effects of the sedative to wear off. You may experience some bloating and gas for a few hours afterward until you expel the injected air. This is not the best time for air travel because the gas may expand and become painful.

Colonoscopy is frequently used for colorectal cancer screening for people at average risk who are age 50 or older.

Sigmoidoscopy

For this procedure, the doctor examines just your rectum and sigmoid colon (and perhaps part of the descending colon) rather than the entire colon. You generally aren't sedated for sigmoidoscopy and the only preparation is typically one or two enemas.

Your doctor may order a sigmoid exam to find the cause of diarrhea, abdominal pain, constipation or bleeding, or to look for signs of cancer. Sigmoidoscopy can be a routine part of cancer screening for people at average risk who are age 50 or older, often combined with a stool test for occult bleeding.

Sigmoidoscopy takes only about 10 to 15 minutes, although it may run longer if your doctor needs to take biopsies or treat inflamed or bleeding tissue. You may experience some bloating for a few hours afterward until you expel the injected air. If polyps are found during a sigmoid exam, the next step is generally a colonoscopy to remove the polyps and to examine the entire colon for additional polyps.

Capsule endoscopy

When endoscopic examinations of your upper and lower gastrointestinal tract are unable to identify the cause of digestive symptoms, your doctor may turn to capsule endoscopy. This test allows the doctor to see areas of your small intestine that are not easily reached with the other procedures.

To start the exam, several adhesive patches are attached to your abdomen. Each patch contains an antenna with wires connected to a recorder that you wear on a belt around your waist.

Then, you swallow a coated capsule, about the size of a vitamin, which contains a minicamera. The camera takes pictures as it travels into your small intestine. These images are collected and stored on the recorder.

The procedure is complete after about eight hours. Over this time, you can participate in many regular activities but your doctor will notify you of certain restrictions. For example, you may be asked to avoid strenuous exercise or any activity that disrupts the recorder. You may drink liquids two hours after the start of the exam, and a light meal after four hours.

The images saved on the recorder are transferred to a computer with special software that strings the images together to create a video. When you see the camera capsule in the toilet after a bowel movement, it may be safely flushed down the toilet.

Capsule endoscopy is most often used to look for sources of gastrointestinal bleeding, such as ulcers or abnormal blood vessels. Sometimes, inflammatory bowel disease as well as polyps and tumors can be diagnosed.

The test cannot be performed on individuals with previous bowel obstruc-tions or narrow areas (strictures) in their intestinal tracts since this might cause the capsule to become stuck.

Endoscopic ultrasound

As the name suggests, endoscopic ultrasound (EUS) combines an endoscopic examination with ultrasound technology. EUS creates images of internal organs using an endoscope that's equipped with both a video camera and an ultrasound probe.

First, an endoscope is positioned within your esophagus, stomach, duodenum, sigmoid colon or rectum. Then, ultrasound waves are emitted from the tip of the scope. The reflected signals are collected and projected on an external monitor, which allows your doctor to closely examine your gastrointestinal tract and nearby organs. EUS also allows your doctor to biopsy abnormal tissue, using ultrasound guidance to pass a fine needle through the stomach or intestinal wall.

As with other endoscopic tests, sedation for endoscopic ultrasound is usually required, as well as monitoring the recovery from sedation. This technology is particularly useful in viewing tumors and other abnormalities of the gastrointestinal tract, allowing for an accurate assessment of tumor spread, if the tumors are malignant. EUS is performed on an outpatient basis and typically takes one to two hours.

Ambulatory acid (pH) probe test

This test helps determine if you have acid reflux, when stomach acid regurgitates into your esophagus and inflames esophageal tissue. Left untreated, this condition leads directly to gastroesophageal reflux disease (GERD).

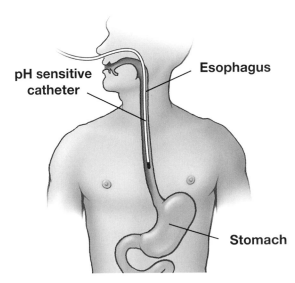

Ambulatory acid pH probe

The test uses an acid-measuring (pH) probe to identify when, and for how long, reflux takes place. Insertion of the probe, attached to the tip of a catheter, takes about 10 minutes. While you're seated, a nurse or technician may spray your throat with a numbing medication before the catheter is threaded through a nasal passage (less frequently, your mouth) and into your esophagus.

The probe is positioned just above the muscular valve (lower esophageal sphincter) between your esophagus and stomach. A second probe may be placed on the catheter in the area of your upper esophagus. The catheter will not interfere with your breathing, and most people experience little or no discomfort during the procedure.

Connected to the other end of the catheter is a small computer that records acid measurements. You wear it around your waist or with a strap over your shoulder during the test. After the device is in place, you may move around and go home.

During the time that monitoring takes place, you will be instructed on when to eat and drink, and you will not be allowed to bathe or go swimming. The following day you return to have the device removed.

Knowing how frequently and for how long periods of acid reflux take place helps your doctor determine how best to treat your problem. This test also can help determine if reflux may be causing other signs and symptoms, such as chest pain, coughing or wheezing, by correlating episodes of acid reflux with their onset. You may be asked to track these signs and symptoms.

An ambulatory acid (pH) probe test is sometimes used to determine if treatment to control acid reflux is working. In addition to probes in your upper and lower esophagus, a third probe may be placed in your stomach to measure the acid level there.

Esophageal muscle test

This test, called manometry, is given if your doctor suspects that you have a swallowing problem caused by esophageal muscles that aren't working properly. During manometry (muh-NOM-uh-tre), a tiny, pressure-sensitive catheter is inserted through your nose (less frequently, your mouth) and into your esophagus. There, it measures muscle pressures as you swallow water.

When you swallow, the muscles in your esophagus normally contract and relax in rolling waves (peristalsis) that propel food and liquid toward your stomach. In addition, muscular valves at the top and bottom of your esophagus (the upper and lower esophageal sphincters) relax and open to let materials pass. They tighten again to protect the sensitive tissue lining the esophagus.

Malfunctions with the muscles in the walls of the esophagus or with the muscular valves can cause difficulty swallowing and lead to gastroesophageal reflux and chest pains. They may also be the cause of pneumonia due to the aspiration of tiny bits of stomach contents into your lungs.

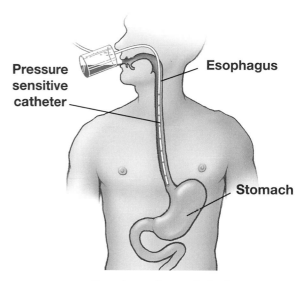

Pressure sensitive catheter

Esophagus

Stomach

Esophageal muscle test

Manometry is most often used after other tests or treatments have failed to identify a problem. The test takes less than an hour. On occasion, manometry may be used to measure pressure in other parts of your digestive tract.

Transit studies

If other diagnostic tests can't determine a cause for persistent abdominal pain, nausea, vomiting, constipation or diarrhea, your doctor may order one of several transit studies. These are tests to measure how quickly food passes through your digestive tract, either in certain parts of the system or in its entirety. If your digestive muscles or nerves aren't working properly, food may move through the tract too quickly or too slowly.

For any of the transit studies that are described below, you cannot be on certain medications, such as narcotics, before having the tests.

Gastric emptying

This test evaluates how quickly your stomach empties food into your small intestine. Your doctor may order this test for unexplained vomiting or if you feel full after eating just a moderate amount of food. For example, if you have diabetes, you could be at risk of gastroparesis (gas-tro-puh-RE-sis), a condition in which your stomach empties too slowly.

You start the test with overnight fasting. At your doctor's office the following day, you consume bread, milk and several eggs. These eggs contain a few drops of a slightly radioactive tracer substance that's clear and tasteless.

After finishing breakfast, you stand or lie on your back while gamma cameras take pictures of the consumed eggs as they pass through your stomach. The pictures don't show your internal organs, only the radioactive tracer element in the eggs.

The first pictures are taken right after you eat, followed by pictures at one hour, two hours and four hours. Each picture session takes about five minutes. Between sessions you can sit or walk around.

Your doctor is aware of the rate at which a normal stomach will empty and, by tracking the movement of the tracer element, can compare it to the rate at which your stomach empties.

Gastric emptying and small bowel transit

This test is similar to the gastric emptying test, except that an additional series of pictures is taken at six hours. If your small intestine is moving the food normally, most of the radioactive eggs will have passed through your small intestine by this time and be in your colon.

Whole gut transit

This test is done if your doctor suspects that the digestive process isn't moving food normally, but he or she is uncertain of where in your gastrointestinal tract the problem is located.

You begin the exam by swallowing a capsule containing a radioactive tracer substance. The capsule is designed to remain intact through the upper digestive tract until it reaches your colon. In the colon, it dissolves and releases the tracer into the lower digestive tract.

About one hour after taking the capsule, you eat the same egg breakfast used in other transit studies, followed by a similar schedule of picture sessions with a gamma camera. This provides a record of how the upper gastrointestinal tract empties.

Whole gut transit study

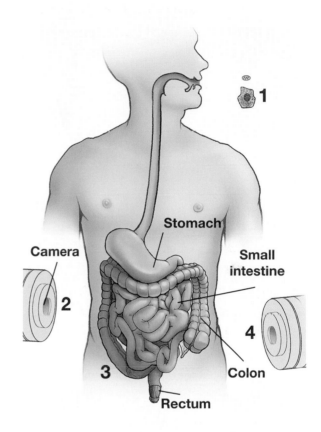

1: Capsule containing tracer is swallowed and egg breakfast is eaten
2: Picture session shows tracer from egg moving through stomach and small intestine
3: Capsule dissolves in colon, releasing tracer pellets
4: Picture session reveals tracer from pellets mixed with food waste moving through colon

An important difference with this exam is that you come back for a picture session about 24 hours after taking the capsule. By this time, the capsule should have released the tracer, which should be seen mixed in with food residue in the middle or lower colon. If the tracer substance remains concentrated in the upper part of your colon, it probably means that the colon isn't propelling food waste normally.

Colonic transit

If you have severe, persistent constipation, your doctor may order a study that focuses only on your colon. You take the same capsule as given in the whole gut transit study but, in this case, you don't need to eat the specially prepared egg breakfast. Instead, a nurse or medical technician will instruct you on the times when you can eat meals throughout the day.

Pictures are taken as soon as you swallow the capsule, then four hours later. By the time of the four-hour picture, the capsule should have reached your upper colon. You will need to return to the office 24 hours later for a picture session to see how far the tracer element has progressed in your colon.

As in the whole gut study, if the tracer element hasn't moved to your middle or lower colon, your colon isn't moving food fast enough. This would help explain your constipation.

Part 2

Digestive diseases

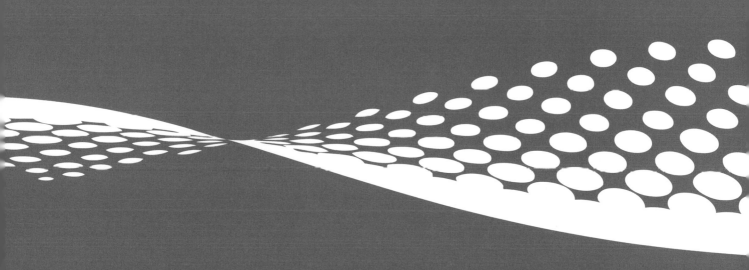

Chapter 5

Gastroesophageal reflux disease (GERD)

Nearly everyone has experienced heartburn, that hot, burning sensation in the middle of your chest, and sometimes in your throat, caused by stomach acid washing back into your esophagus. It may be because you ate too much at dinner. Or perhaps you didn't let a bedtime snack digest before you laid down for the night.

Key signs and symptoms

- Heartburn
- Acid reflux
- Difficulty swallowing
- Chest pain
- Persistent coughing
- Hoarseness

Heartburn is common, and an occasional episode is generally nothing to worry about. Many people, however, battle heartburn regularly, even daily. About 20 percent of Americans have heartburn weekly, and many have it every day. Frequent or constant heartburn can be a serious problem and deserves medical attention. Most often, it's a symptom of gastroesophageal reflux disease (GERD).

What's GERD?

After you chew and swallow, a soft, rounded mass of food, or bolus, travels down your esophagus to the muscular valve that separates your esophagus from your stomach.

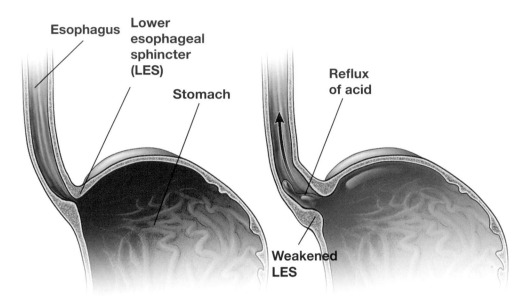

Normally, the lower esophageal sphincter (LES) remains closed, preventing stomach acid from washing up into the esophagus (image at left). If the LES becomes weakened or relaxed, acid can reflux into the esophagus, causing heartburn and tissue inflammation (image at right).

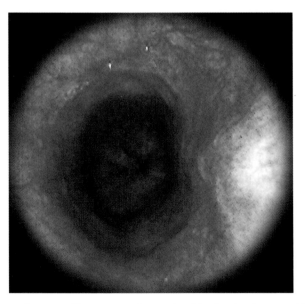
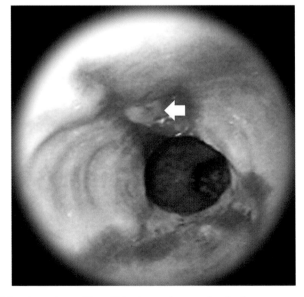

A normal lower esophageal sphincter is shown at left in closed position. Weakened muscles in the sphincter at right can no longer close the esophagus, allowing continued backflow of digestive juices. Inflammation and linear ulcers (arrow) extend up the esophageal walls.

Called the lower esophageal sphincter (LES), this valve opens to allow the bolus to pass into your stomach and then closes tightly again.

If the valve weakens or closes abnormally, it doesn't close as tightly as it should. Stomach acid washes back into your lower esophagus through the opening. The flowing back of stomach acid is known as reflux. It can cause frequent heartburn and disrupt daily life.

Stomach acid also may regurgitate higher to your upper esophagus, leaving a sour taste in your mouth or causing you to cough.

A constant backwash of acid can irritate the lining of the esophagus, causing inflammation (esophagitis). Over time, the inflammation may erode the lining of the esophagus, causing an open sore to form (esophageal ulcer) that may bleed and cause pain. Damage to the lining can also lead to the formation of scar tissue, which narrows the food pathway and makes swallowing difficult. Changes in the color and composition of the esophageal lining from reflux are associated with a higher risk of esophageal cancer.

Gastroesophageal reflux disease is the name for chronic acid reflux that causes esophagitis or other complications. Anyone can have GERD — even children and infants. Studies show that GERD is no more common in older adults than in younger adults. However, its signs and symptoms may be more severe in older adults.

Other causes of esophagitis

The most common cause of an inflamed esophagus (esophagitis) is GERD, but esophagitis can have other causes. A fungus or virus can inflame esophageal tissue, especially in people with weakened immune systems, for example, individuals with diabetes or on corticosteroid medication. Certain pills also may irritate tissue during swallowing (pill esophagitis), especially if taken without adequate liquid or while lying down. These include the antibiotics erythromycin and tetracycline, alendronate (Fosamax) taken for osteoporosis, vitamin C tablets, iron, and potassium.

Variation in signs and symptoms

Acid reflux and heartburn are two problems that most people with GERD will share. Other signs and symptoms may be present but what they are usually varies from among the following:

Difficulty swallowing

Swallowing problems may indicate a narrowing (stricture) of the esophagus or an inflammation of the esophagus that limits the organ's ability to propel food toward the stomach. In severe cases, you may choke or feel as if food is lodged behind your breastbone.

Coughing

Some people experience a chronic cough with GERD, which may be due to nerve irritation from stomach acid reflux in the esophagus or from small amounts of acid regurgitating into lung airways (bronchi).

Wheezing

If acid reflux appears to worsen, it may cause wheezing that can resemble the symptoms of asthma.

Throat problems

Acid reflux and inflammation may produce hoarseness, a need to keep clearing your throat, a feeling of a lump in your throat (globus sensation), a chronic sore throat or hiccups.

Bleeding

The inflammation and erosion of esophageal lining or the formation of an esophageal ulcer can cause bleeding. The blood may be bright red or darker in color (even black) and appear in vomit or mixed in with stool.

Chest pain

The pain is often worse after a heavy meal or at night. Because GERD and heart disease can coexist, have chest pain evaluated to make sure it's not associated with a heart condition.

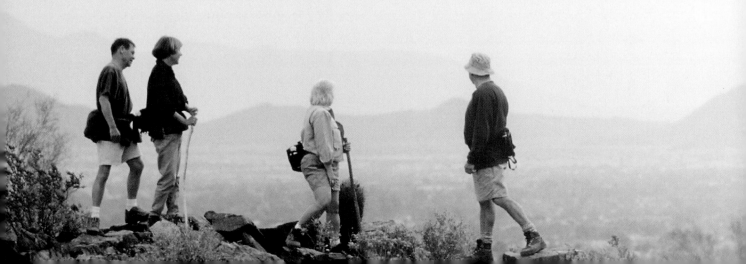

Who gets GERD?

It isn't always easy to pinpoint the cause of GERD. Some people with the disease lack common risk factors that might trigger the problem. Many people, though, have at least one of the following factors that can significantly increase their risk of GERD.

Hiatal hernia
This condition occurs when part of your stomach protrudes into your lower chest, and your diaphragm — the large muscle that separates your chest and abdomen — is no longer able to support the lower esophageal sphincter (see "What's a hiatal hernia" on page 111). Acid reflux increases because of the weakened valve.

Certain foods
Chocolate, fats and mint may contribute to or aggravate GERD. Chemicals in these foods cause the lower esophageal sphincter to relax and open for acid reflux. Caffeine products can increase the amount of stomach acid, which may worsen GERD.

Being overweight
Many, but not all, people with GERD are overweight. Excess weight puts extra pressure on your stomach and diaphragm, which can force open the lower esophageal sphincter. Eating very large meals or meals high in fat may have similar effects.

Excessive alcohol
Alcohol reduces pressure on the lower esophageal sphincter, allowing it to relax and open. Alcohol may also irritate the lining of the esophagus.

Smoking
Smoking may increase the production of stomach acid, aggravating reflux.

Family history
Mayo Clinic researchers believe that a genetic link may predispose some people to the disease. If your parents or siblings have or had GERD, your chances of also developing the condition are increased.

Other conditions or diseases can aggravate or precipitate symptoms of GERD, although they're generally not considered a cause of GERD.

Pregnancy
GERD is more common during pregnancy because of increased production of progesterone. This hormone relaxes many muscles, including the lower esophageal sphincter. GERD during pregnancy may also occur because of increased pressure on the stomach.

Asthma

GERD is more common in people who have asthma, although it's uncertain if asthma is a cause or an effect. One theory is that the coughing and sneezing that accompany asthma may lead to pressure changes in your chest and abdomen, causing the regurgitation of stomach acid into your esophagus. Some asthma medications used to widen (dilate) airways also may relax the lower esophageal sphincter, allowing acid reflux.

It's possible that GERD may worsen asthma symptoms. For example, you may inhale (aspirate) small amounts of digestive juices into your lungs that first were regurgitated into your esophagus. This damages your lung airways.

Diabetes

One complication of diabetes is a disorder in which your stomach takes too long to empty (gastroparesis). When stomach contents remain for too long, they can reflux into the esophagus.

Peptic stomach ulcer

An open sore (ulcer) located near the valve separating your stomach from your small intestine (pylorus, or pyloric valve) can obstruct or hinder valve function. Food and fluid don't empty as fast as they should, causing acid buildup in your stomach and triggering reflux into the esophagus.

Delayed stomach emptying

Abnormal nerve or muscle function in the stomach also can delay emptying and cause acid backup.

Connective tissue disorders

Diseases that cause muscular tissue to thicken and swell, such as scleroderma, can prevent digestive muscles from relaxing and contracting as they should, causing acid reflux.

Zollinger-Ellison syndrome

One complication of this rare disorder is that your stomach produces high amounts of stomach acid, increasing your risk of reflux and GERD.

Danger of inaction

When left untreated, persistent acid reflux can lead to one or more of these common complications of GERD.

Esophageal narrowing

Esophageal narrowing (stricture) occurs in about 10 percent of people with GERD. Exposure to stomach acid damages the cells lining the inner surface of the lower esophagus (reflux esophagitis), leading to the formation of scar tissue. This narrows the esophageal opening through which food must pass to reach the stomach. Scar tissue obstructs chunks of food in the stricture and interferes with swallowing.

Treatment for esophageal narrowing generally consists of an endoscopic procedure that stretches and widens the esophageal passage and an acid-suppressing medication to help prevent the passage from re-narrowing.

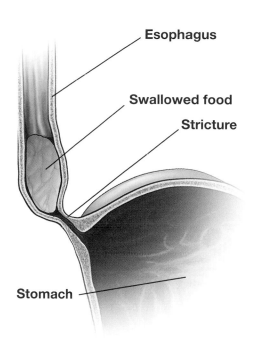

A stricture of the esophagus often prevents swallowed food from reaching the stomach.

Esophageal ulcer

An open sore may form where the reflux of stomach acid severely erodes tissue in the esophageal walls. The ulcer may be painful, bleed and make swallowing difficult. Medications and lifestyle changes to control stomach acid reflux gives damaged tissue time to heal and help cure the ulcer. See Chapter 6 for more information on peptic ulcers.

Barrett's esophagus

Barrett's esophagus is a serious complication of GERD. Although the condition is still uncommon, the number of new cases is increasing.

Changes in the color and composition of tissue lining the lower esophagus signal the development of this condition. Instead of being pink, the tissue turns a salmon color. Instead of finding normal, flat tile-shaped cells (similar to skin cells), a microscopic examination of Barrett's tissue reveals tall cells that resemble the surface of a shag carpet (similar to cells lining the inner surface of the small intestine). This cellular change is called metaplasia — the abnormal replacement of one type of cell for another type.

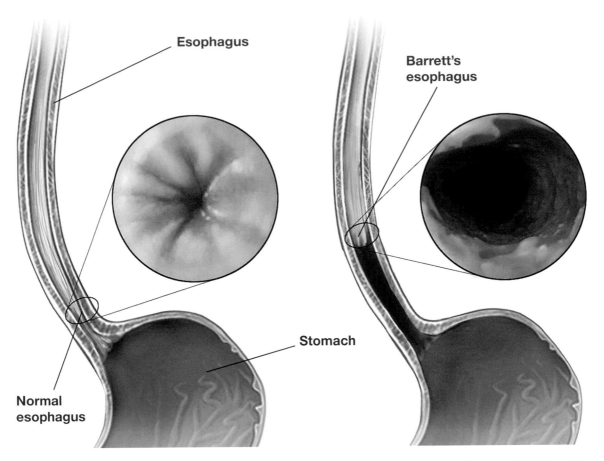

Esophagus

Barrett's esophagus

Stomach

Normal esophagus

The image at left shows the color and compostion of tissue in a normal esophagus. With Barrett's esophagus, in the image at right, a change has taken place in the size, shape and composition of cells lining the esophagus, caused possibly by long-term exposure to acid reflux.

Metaplasia is brought on by repeated and long-term exposure of the esophagus to stomach acid, and the change is associated with a higher risk of getting esophageal cancer. Between 5 and 15 percent of people with GERD have Barrett's esophagus. Once you have it, your chances of developing esophageal cancer are 30 to 125 times as high as that of the general population.

Here's a more positive view of this risk: It's also a fact that most people with Barrett's esophagus do not develop cancer. Thus, the risk of someone with GERD getting cancer remains low.

Endoscopy is the most common procedure for identifying Barrett's esophagus (see pages 84-85). A tiny camera on the endoscope allows your doctor to directly examine your esophagus for tissue damage. Your doctor may remove small pieces of tissue (biopsy) from the lower esophagus and have them examined for evidence of precancerous cellular changes (dysplasia).

The degree of precancerous change in Barrett's esophagus ranges from none, to small but noticeable changes (low-grade dysplasia), to extensive changes (high-grade dysplasia), and finally, to invasive cancer. The more extensive the change, the greater the risk that cancer is present or will develop.

Treatment is available for Barrett's esophagus, but people often go to the doctor when it's too late, after cancer is already present. Treatment typically begins by controlling GERD through diet and lifestyle changes and, often, by taking medications to control acid reflux. Your doctor may recommend periodic endoscopic examinations to monitor the changes.

High-grade dysplasia may be a precursor esophageal cancer. Treatment may involve surgery to remove part of the esophagus. Other options may involve burning away damaged tissue with a high-frequency electrical current (radiofrequency ablation) or heat-producing light (photodynamic therapy).

See your doctor

If you experience heartburn at least twice a week for several weeks, or your symptoms seem to be getting worse, it would be prudent to see your doctor and discuss your concerns.

At the initial visit, your doctor may ask about your general health and about the signs and symptoms you're experiencing. When did you notice them starting? How often do they occur? Are they becoming more severe? Do certain factors, for example, a type of activity or food, seem to make your signs and symptoms better or worse?

Your doctor may also ask questions about your lifestyle. Do you smoke? What are your eating habits? Have you gained weight recently? How much alcohol do you drink?

If you have the typical signs and symptoms of GERD — heartburn and acid reflux — and you don't have additional problems, you may not need any diagnostic tests. However, if your heartburn is severe or you have additional signs and symptoms including unexplained weight loss or difficulty with swallowing (dysphagia), you'll probably need some testing before your doctor can make a diagnosis.

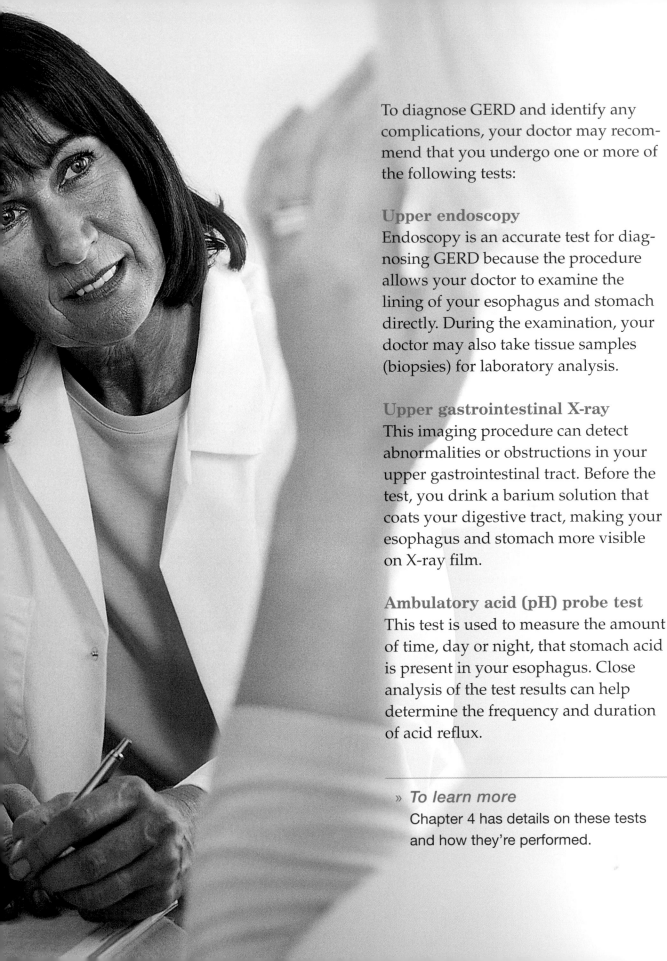

To diagnose GERD and identify any complications, your doctor may recommend that you undergo one or more of the following tests:

Upper endoscopy

Endoscopy is an accurate test for diagnosing GERD because the procedure allows your doctor to examine the lining of your esophagus and stomach directly. During the examination, your doctor may also take tissue samples (biopsies) for laboratory analysis.

Upper gastrointestinal X-ray

This imaging procedure can detect abnormalities or obstructions in your upper gastrointestinal tract. Before the test, you drink a barium solution that coats your digestive tract, making your esophagus and stomach more visible on X-ray film.

Ambulatory acid (pH) probe test

This test is used to measure the amount of time, day or night, that stomach acid is present in your esophagus. Close analysis of the test results can help determine the frequency and duration of acid reflux.

» *To learn more*
Chapter 4 has details on these tests and how they're performed.

Treatment starts with self-care

Regardless of the severity of your signs and symptoms, the first step in managing GERD is to assess your behaviors and lifestyle. To control mild signs and symptoms, slight changes to your daily routine might be at least part of what's needed to manage the disease. To handle severe signs and symptoms, more profound lifestyle changes and medication may make your condition easier to control.

Stop smoking
Smoking increases acid reflux and can dry up saliva. Saliva helps to protect your esophagus from stomach acid.

Eat smaller meals
Smaller portions at meals reduce the pressure on your lower esophageal sphincter. Too much pressure can force the valve open, allowing acid reflux.

Allow time to digest
Wait at least three hours before lying down to sleep or nap. By then, most of the food in your stomach will have emptied into the small intestine. Don't exercise immediately after a meal. Wait two to three hours before engaging in strenuous physical activity.

Limit fatty foods
Studies show a potentially strong link between the consumption of fat and GERD. Fatty foods relax the esophageal sphincter, permitting stomach acid to flow into the esophagus. Fat also slows stomach emptying, increasing the time acid can regurgitate into the esophagus.

Avoid problem foods
Foods and beverages such as onions, spicy foods, chocolate, mint and caffeinated drinks tend to increase stomach acid. Chocolate and mint may relax the lower esophageal sphincter. Acidic foods, such as citrus fruits and tomato-based products, can irritate an inflamed esophagus, making GERD symptoms worse in some people.

If your lower esophageal sphincter is moderately to severely weakened, it doesn't matter what you eat or drink. Stomach acid backs up into your esophagus regardless of stomach contents.

Limit or avoid alcohol
Alcohol relaxes the lower esophageal sphincter and may irritate the esophageal lining, worsening symptoms.

Lose excess weight
Heartburn and acid reflux are more likely to occur when there's added pressure on your stomach from excess

weight. Keep in mind that not everyone with heartburn and GERD will improve after losing weight.

Raise the head of your bed
Raising the head of your bed 3 to 6 inches provides a gradual decline from your head to your feet and helps prevent stomach acid from flowing back into your esophagus while you sleep. The best way to do this is by placing blocks of wood or other sturdy materials under the legs at the head of your bed. Using bigger (or more) pillows to raise your head may worsen acid reflux or cause a neck ache.

Avoid tightfitting clothes
A tight or constricting fit can put more pressure on your stomach.

Take time to relax
Stress can slow digestion and worsen GERD symptoms. Although not scientifically proved, relaxation techniques, such as meditation and yoga, may improve GERD by reducing stress.

Medications can help

Perhaps you've tried many options. You've cut back on fatty foods, ate smaller meals and lost some weight. You've even stopped smoking. Yet your GERD symptoms continue to bother you or have improved very little. When lifestyle changes aren't effective, the next step may be medication.

Antacids

These over-the-counter medications are best suited for occasional or mild heartburn. Antacids neutralize stomach acid for temporary relief. Products have different neutralizing agents. For example, Tums and Rolaids are chewable tablets containing calcium carbonate. Mylanta and Maalox come in liquid or tablet form containing magnesium. Liquids generally work faster than do tablets, but some people find them less convenient.

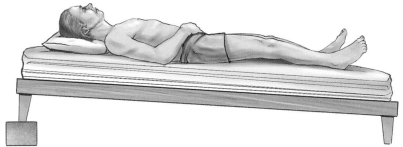

Raising the head slightly above the foot of your bed 3 to 6 inches helps prevent acid reflux.

Drugs and supplements that can worsen GERD

Some medications and supplements may aggravate symptoms of GERD by reducing pressure in the lower esophageal sphincter — allowing the muscular valve to relax — or by irritating the esophageal lining. If you're bothered by GERD, try to avoid the following medications or supplements, if possible. If you're already taking one or more of these medications, talk with your doctor first before you stop taking it. Sudden stoppage could be dangerous to your health.

- Anticholinergics — medications that relax smooth muscle
- Calcium channel blockers — medications for high blood pressure
- Potassium tablets
- Vitamin C tablets
- Tetracycline — antibiotic in capsule form
- Nonsteroidal anti-inflammatory drugs (NSAIDs), such as aspirin, ibuprofen (Advil, Motrin, others), naproxen (Aleve) and ketoprofen
- Quinidine — heart-arrhythmia medication
- Sedatives and tranquilizers
- Alendronate (Fosamax) — osteoporosis medication

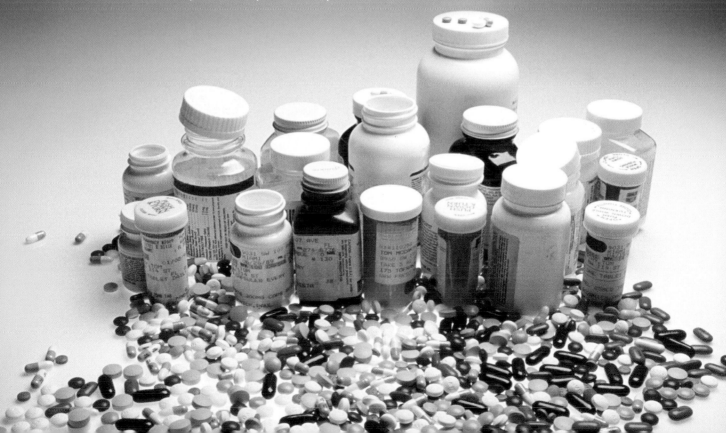

Antacids can relieve signs and symptoms, but they won't cure the cause of acid reflux. The products are generally safe, but if taken frequently they can produce certain side effects, such as diarrhea (especially magnesium-containing antacids), constipation (especially aluminum-containing antacids) or congestive heart failure (especially sodium-containing antacids).

Some antacids may also interact with other medications, including medications for kidney or heart disease. Constant use of products containing magnesium may cause a magnesium buildup, which can aggravate or result in kidney disease, especially if you have diabetes. Too much calcium can result in kidney stones. If you take an antacid regularly, discuss these concerns with your doctor.

Acid blockers

Also known as histamine (H-2) blockers, these popular medications are available over-the-counter and by prescription. Instead of neutralizing gastric acid, they reduce the amount of acid produced in your stomach.

Acid blockers differ from antacids in that they can prevent acid reflux and heartburn, not just relieve it. They're also longer acting, relieving heartburn for up to 12 hours, rather than four hours or less for antacids.

Acid blockers include cimetidine (Tagamet), famotidine (Pepcid), nizatidine (Axid) and ranitidine (Zantac). The over-the-counter acid blockers are about half the strength of their prescription counterparts.

It's best to take acid blockers before any meal that may give you heartburn. You can take them after the symptoms occur, of course, but it takes about 30 minutes before they take effect.

Acid blockers help heal inflammation (esophagitis) and ulcers by reducing the exposure of esophageal tissues to stomach acid. Your doctor may recommend that you take an acid blocker for several months, or longer, if it helps to keep your symptoms at bay.

These medications are generally safe but can infrequently cause side effects, including diarrhea, constipation, dry mouth, dizziness and drowsiness. Some acid blockers, especially cimetidine, carry the risk of dangerous interactions with other medications. Check with your doctor or pharmacist about possible drug interactions.

What's a hiatal hernia?

If the upper portion of your stomach protrudes into your lower chest cavity, it forms a pocket that's known as a hiatal hernia. A hiatal hernia was once thought to be the most common cause of gastroesophageal reflux disease, but doctors now take a different view. Only moderate to large hiatal hernias seem to play a role in GERD — either by contributing to severe acid reflux or by aggravating existing GERD symptoms.

Your chest cavity and abdomen are separated by a large, dome-shaped muscle called the diaphragm. A small opening (hiatus) in the diaphragm allows the esophagus to pass through to the stomach. A hiatal hernia forms when the upper stomach pushes upward through the hiatus into the cavity above the diaphragm.

Esophagus

Lower esophageal sphincter

Hiatal hernia

Diaphragm

With a hiatal hernia, the upper stomach protrudes above the diaphragm.

A small hiatal hernia isn't likely to cause problems. In fact, most hiatal hernias cause no signs and symptoms at all. Moderate or large hernias can contribute to heartburn in one of two ways. Normally, your diaphragm is aligned with your lower esophageal sphincter, supporting and providing pressure on the sphincter to keep it closed. The hiatal hernia displaces the sphincter into the chest cavity, thereby reducing pressure on the valve and allowing it to open. A hiatal hernia can also cause heartburn if it becomes a reservoir for stomach acid, which can travel up the esophagus.

Pain, bloating, difficulty swallowing or obstruction of your esophagus may occur if the portion of the stomach that protrudes into the chest cavity becomes twisted. In rare cases, a large portion of your stomach may protrude into the chest cavity, restricting blood flow to the stomach. This can produce severe chest pain and difficulty swallowing. Large hiatal hernias that pose these kinds of problems are generally treated with surgery. The procedure returns the stomach to its normal position, realigning the diaphragm and lower esophageal sphincter, and restoring pressure on the sphincter to keep it closed.

Proton pump inhibitors (PPIs)

These medications are the most effective for treatment of GERD. Dexlansoprazole (Dexilant), esomeprazole (Nexium), lansoprazole (Prevacid), omeprazole (Prilosec), omeprazole-sodium bicarbonate (Zegerid), pantoprazole (Protonix) and rabeprazole (Aciphex) are available by prescription. Omeprazole (Prilosec OTC) and lansoprazole (Prevacid 24HR) are available over-the-counter.

PPIs block the production of gastric acid and allow time for damaged esophageal tissue to heal. PPIs are convenient to use because you generally take them only once a day. However, the drugs are more expensive than other GERD medications.

PPIs are generally safe and well tolerated for long-term treatment of GERD. In trials, PPIs have been found safe to use for up to at least 10 years. If your GERD is severe, your doctor may recommend the drugs for indefinite use to keep your symptoms under control.

Side effects may occur in a small number of people taking PPIs. These side effects may include stomach or abdominal pain, diarrhea, constipation, headache, or lightheadedness. If the side effects are mild, your dosage may not require an adjustment or possible discontinuation. The drugs may be used in combination with H-2 blockers in people who experience acid reflux symptoms at night.

It's important to take your PPI about 15 to 30 minutes before a meal. These medications are far less effective if taken while you're fasting.

When surgery may be needed

Because of the effectiveness of medications for treatment in both the short term and the long term, using surgery to treat GERD is uncommon. However, surgery may become an option if you can't tolerate the medications, if the medications are ineffective, or if you can't afford the cost of drugs in long-term use.

Your doctor may also recommend surgery if you have any of the following complications:

- Large hiatal hernia (see "What's a hiatal hernia?" on page 111)

- Severe esophagitis, especially with bleeding
- Recurrent narrowing (stricture) of the esophagus
- Barrett's esophagus, especially with progressive precancerous or cancerous changes
- Severe pulmonary problems, such as bronchitis or pneumonia, due to acid reflux

Before 1991, an open surgical procedure known as Nissen fundoplication was the surgery of choice for severe GERD. Today, doctors perform the same surgery with similar success by using laparoscopy — the surgeon works through a few small abdominal incisions instead of a single large one. The advantages of laparoscopic surgery are shorter recovery time and less discomfort.

Nissen fundoplication involves tightening the lower esophageal sphincter to prevent acid reflux. This is accomplished by wrapping the very top of your stomach around the outside of the lower esophagus. The surgery takes about two hours and typically requires a one- or two-day hospital stay.

During laparoscopic surgery, the surgeon generally makes three to four tiny incisions in your abdomen and inserts small instruments through the incisions, including an endoscope equipped with a tiny camera to see the procedure. To provide more space for your surgeon to work, your abdomen is inflated with carbon dioxide.

Most people who undergo Nissen fundoplication remain free of GERD symptoms for at least one year. In one study, almost 90 percent were symptom-free after five years. These success rates apply equally to the laparoscopic and open procedures.

Other surgical procedures for GERD include Toupet fundoplication, Hill repair and the Belsey Mark IV operation. All involve restructuring the lower esophageal sphincter to improve its strength and ability to prevent reflux. These surgeries are done less often, and their success is often dependent on the skill and experience of the surgeon.

Complications from any of the surgical procedures for GERD generally are mild, but may include difficulty swallowing, bloating, diarrhea and a sense of feeling full after eating only a moderate amount — a sensation known as early satiety.

Chapter 6

Ulcers and stomach pain

Too much stress, too much spicy food, and it was thought that you could be headed for an ulcer. Not long ago, the common belief was that ulcers were a direct result of how you lived your life. That burning pain in your chest was the outcome, for example, of you dealing with the pressures of an intense, fast-paced job or eating too much of the kinds of food that were poorly suited to your digestive tract.

A great deal has changed in recent decades. Doctors now know that most ulcers are the result of a bacterial infection or a medication, not of lifestyle factors. Accordingly, your treatment options are very different now from what they used to be. Instead of taking months or years to treat, ulcers can often be cured in two to eight weeks.

Key signs and symptoms

- Gnawing pain in stomach or upper abdomen
- Blood in vomit
- Blood in stool
- Unexplained weight loss
- Pain in the midback

There's one small catch. Some people who think they have ulcers really don't. Instead, they may have a condition called nonulcer dyspepsia (dis-PEP-see-uh), in which symptoms may mimic those of an ulcer. Unlike ulcers, which are decreasing in number, the reported cases of nonulcer dyspepsia appear to be on the rise.

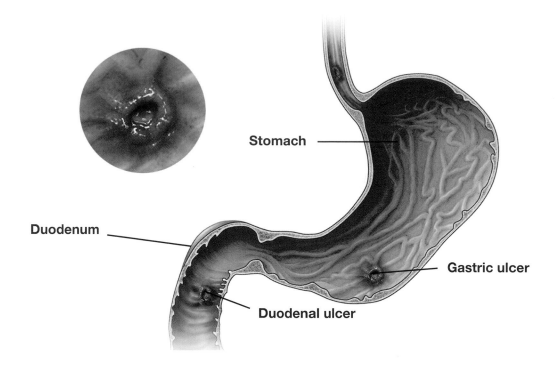

Stomach

Duodenum

Gastric ulcer

Duodenal ulcer

A peptic ulcer is a sore in the lining of your stomach or small intestine. A peptic ulcer located in your stomach is called a gastric ulcer. A peptic ulcer in the small intestine most often occurs in the uppermost part, or duodenum, and is called a duodenal ulcer.

An open sore

Ulcer is the medical term for an open sore on your body. There are several types of ulcers. One is a pressure ulcer (bedsore, or decubitus ulcer) that can occur on your back or buttocks from lying too long in one position. Another is a stasis ulcer that can develop on an ankle from obstructed blood flow.

The most common type of ulcer — and the type that people generally associate with the term *ulcer* — is a peptic ulcer.

Peptic ulcers develop on the inside lining of the stomach or small intestine. About 10 percent of Americans will experience a peptic ulcer at some point in life.

A peptic ulcer that occurs in your stomach is called a gastric ulcer. If the ulcer develops in your small intestine, it's named for the section of the intestine where it's located. The most common is a duodenal (doo-o-DEE-nul) ulcer, because the sore develops in the duodenum, which is the first, or uppermost, part of the small intestine.

Left untreated, peptic ulcers can cause internal bleeding and create a hole in the wall of your stomach or small intestine, putting you at risk of serious inflammation or infection in your abdominal cavity (peritonitis). Peptic ulcers can also cause scar tissue to develop. Scarring can obstruct the passage of food through the digestive tract and result in weight loss.

The most common symptom of a peptic ulcer is a gnawing pain in your upper abdomen between your navel and breastbone (sternum). This pain, caused by stomach acid washing over the open sore, may linger for just a few minutes, or it may last for hours.

The pain from an ulcer is often worse when your stomach is empty — and therefore the pain tends to flare at night. In contrast, food helps buffer the acid. That's why eating often temporarily relieves the pain. Some people with ulcers experience weight gain because pain leads them to eat more often.

Other signs and symptoms of peptic ulcers include vomiting blood, which may appear bright red or black like coffee grounds, and producing stools that are discolored by dark-colored blood. Ulcers may also produce pain in the midback region.

Bacteria are common culprits

A major breakthrough in the understanding and treatment of peptic ulcers occurred in 1983 when two Australian researchers noticed corkscrew-shaped bacteria in biopsy specimens of people who had ulcers and persistent stomach inflammation (gastritis).

The bacteria discovered by the researchers, called Helicobacter pylori (*H. pylori* or *HP*), live and multiply within the mucous layer that covers and protects tissues lining the stomach and, sometimes, the upper part of the duodenum. Often, *H. pylori* causes no problems. But sometimes it can erode digestive tissues, producing an ulcer. Approximately 1 in 5 people infected with *H. pylori* gets an ulcer.

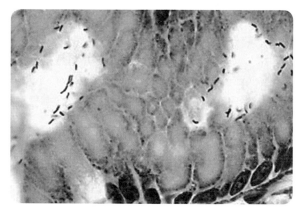

This sample reveals *H. pylori* bacteria in the mucous layer overlying stomach tissue.

Although it's not clear how the organisms spread, they appear to be transmitted from person to person by direct contact with saliva or fecal matter. Children sharing beds, poor food handling and substandard sanitation practices are thought to be common routes of transmission. Because scientists have found *H. pylori* in water, they suspect the infection may also be transmitted in contaminated drinking water.

The stomach and its stomach acid make a hostile environment for many bacteria. But *H. pylori* is well-adapted for survival in the stomach. It produces an enzyme that creates a buffer zone to resist the acid.

Risk factors for peptic ulcers include:

- Being born in a developing country
- Having a low socioeconomic standard of living
- Living in a large family or in crowded conditions
- Being exposed to the vomit of an infected individual

The good news is that the rate of new infection from *H. pylori* seems to be dropping in the United States. American children raised in the 1920s to the 1940s were much more likely to have been infected than are today's children.

About 50 percent of people older than 60 have *H. pylori*, while only about 20 percent of Americans under the age of 40 are infected with it.

Major factors that may have contributed to the decrease in *H. pylori* infection are overall improvements among the general population in socioeconomic status and in public hygiene and sanitation.

Another change is the widespread use of antibiotics in children. Treating conditions such as ear infections and other common childhood illnesses with antibiotics may have done double duty by also preventing or treating *H. pylori* infection early in life.

Other causes of ulcers

H. pylori is the most common, but not the only, cause of peptic ulcers. *H. pylori* presently accounts for about two-thirds of all peptic ulcers in the United States. The rate of *H. pylori* infection is higher in areas of high population density and poverty, and lower in areas of low population density and with a higher standard of living.

Besides *H. pylori*, other causes of peptic ulcers include:

Regular use of pain relievers

Nonsteroidal anti-inflammatory drugs (NSAIDs) can irritate or inflame the lining of your stomach and small intestine. To help avoid this upset, many people take NSAIDs with meals.

Between 15 and 30 percent of people who regularly take NSAIDs develop ulcers. The drugs inhibit the production of an enzyme that produces prostaglandins — hormone-like substances that protect your stomach lining. Without this protection, stomach acid erodes the lining, causing bleeding and ulcers. Regular use of NSAIDs may also increase ulcer risk in people already infected with *H. pylori* bacteria.

NSAIDs are available both by prescription and over-the-counter. Non-prescription forms include aspirin, ibuprofen (Advil, Motrin, others), naproxen (Aleve) and ketoprofen.

The pain reliever acetaminophen (Tylenol, others) doesn't inhibit the production of prostaglandins and doesn't cause stomach ulcers.

Smoking

Nicotine, the primary active ingredient in tobacco, increases the volume and concentration of gastric acid in your stomach — which increases your risk of an ulcer. Tobacco use may also slow the healing process during ulcer treatment.

Excessive alcohol consumption

Alcohol can irritate and erode the mucous lining of your stomach and intestines, causing inflammation and bleeding. It's uncertain, however, whether this development alone can progress into an ulcer or whether other contributing factors must be present, such as *H. pylori* bacteria or nicotine.

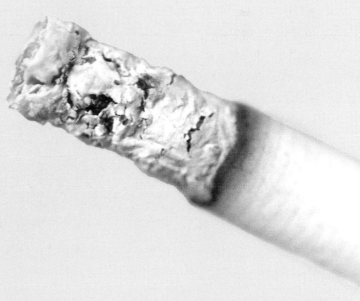

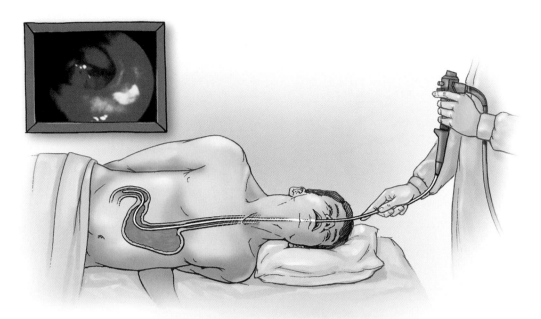

If a peptic ulcer may be causing symptoms, your doctor may perform an upper gastrointestinal endoscopy to examine your stomach and upper part of the small intestine (duodenum). Images appear on an external monitor as your doctor guides the endoscope through your digestive tract.

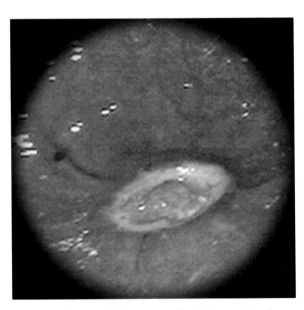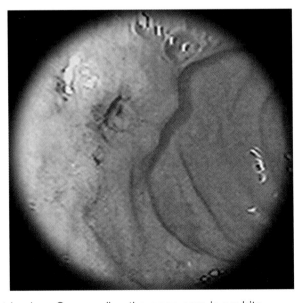

The endoscopic image on the left reveals a large gastric ulcer. Surrounding the open sore is a white ring consisting of dead tissue and debris. The endoscopic image on the right shows a duodenal ulcer, with a deep, flat, pigmented base at the center with thick margins of tissue.

Diagnosing ulcers

If a peptic ulcer is suspected, your doctor may begin the diagnostic procedure with an upper gastrointestinal (GI) X-ray of your stomach and duodenum. (For more on this procedure, see page 79.) Before the X-ray, you swallow barium, a thick, white liquid that coats your digestive tract, making an ulcer more visible on the image. This test can detect some ulcers, but not all.

Endoscopy may follow if the upper GI X-ray suggests a possible ulcer — or your doctor may simply choose to perform upper gastrointestinal endoscopy in place of an X-ray. (For more on this procedure, see pages 84-85.)

Endoscopy is a more sensitive procedure than an X-ray. The flexible tube with attached camera (endoscope) is threaded down your throat into your stomach and duodenum. This instrument allows your doctor to examine your upper digestive tract via images relayed to an external monitor.

If an ulcer is found, your doctor may remove small tissue samples (biopsy) near the ulcer. These samples are examined under a microscope to rule out stomach cancer. (Cancer of the duodenum is rare, so a biopsy of a duodenal ulcer is seldom necessary.) A biopsy can also identify the presence of *H. pylori* in your stomach lining.

In addition to a biopsy, three other tests can determine if the cause of your ulcer is *H. pylori* infection:

Blood test

This test checks for *H. pylori* antibodies in your system. Unfortunately, test results don't distinguish between past and current infections. After the bacteria have been eradicated, you may still show positive results.

Breath test

To start this test, you blow into a small plastic bag that is immediately sealed. Then, you drink a glass of liquid with a substance containing a radioactive carbon atom. Later, you blow into a second bag. If you're infected with *H. pylori*, the second breath sample will contain the radioactive carbon broken down into carbon dioxide by the bacteria. It takes a day to get test results.

If you're taking a proton pump inhibitor (PPI), you'll need to stop taking the medication for at least two weeks before the test because PPIs interfere with test results. Taking antibiotics or bismuth subsalicylate (Pepto-Bismol) also interferes with test results.

Ulcers that fail to heal

Approximately 90 percent of all peptic ulcers heal within six to eight weeks. Those that don't are called refractory ulcers. There are many reasons why an ulcer may fail to heal. Not taking medications according to directions is one reason. Another is that some types of *H. pylori* are resistant to antibiotic drugs. Other factors that can interfere with the healing process include regular use of tobacco, alcohol or nonsteroidal anti-inflammatory drugs (NSAIDs). Sometimes, the problem is accidental — people are unaware that a medication they're taking contains an NSAID.

In rare cases, refractory ulcers may be a result of extreme overproduction of stomach acid, an infection other than *H. pylori*, or the development of other digestive diseases, including Crohn's disease or cancer. Some people develop ulcers without any known reason for getting them.

Treatment for refractory ulcers generally involves eliminating certain factors that may interfere with healing, along with prescribing stronger doses of ulcer-healing medications. Sometimes, new medications may be added to the initial combination. Surgery to help heal an ulcer may be necessary only when the ulcer doesn't respond to aggressive drug treatment.

The breath test is comparable in accuracy to the blood test. The advantage of the breath test is how it monitors the effectiveness of treatment to eradicate *H. pylori* — it quickly detects when the bacteria have been killed in your digestive tract. With the blood test, *H. pylori* antibodies may still be present a year or more after the infection is gone, giving you false positive test results.

Stool antigen test

This test checks for *H. pylori* in stool samples, indicating possible infection in your digestive tract. The test may also help monitor successful treatment. Taking proton pump inhibitors, antibiotics or bismuth subsalicylate (Pepto-Bismol) can interfere with test results and should be discontinued four to six weeks before the stool test.

Treatment combinations

Over-the-counter antacids and acid blockers may help relieve the gnawing pain of an ulcer, but your relief will always be short-lived. A peptic ulcer isn't something you should attempt to treat solely on your own.

With a doctor's help, you can find prompt relief from ulcer pain as well as a lifelong cure from the disease. Because most ulcers stem from *H. pylori* bacteria, doctors use a two-pronged approach to treatment:

- Kill the bacteria
- Reduce the amount of acid in your digestive tract to help relieve pain and encourage healing

Accomplishing two steps requires use of at least three — and sometimes four — of the following medications:

Antibiotics

Different combinations of antibiotics with proton pump inhibitors or bismuth subsalicylate (Pepto-Bismol) or both can kill *H. pylori* most of the time. For any of the combination treatments to work, you should try to follow your doctor's instructions precisely.

The antibiotics most commonly prescribed for treatment of *H. pylori* include amoxicillin, clarithromycin (Biaxin), metronidazole (Flagyl) and tetracycline. Some pharmaceutical companies package a combination of two antibiotics together, with an acid suppressor or cytoprotective agent specifically developed for treatment of *H. pylori* infection. These combination treatments are sold under the names Prevpac and Helidac.

You'll need to take the antibiotic combination for only one to two weeks, depending on the type and number of medications your doctor prescribes. Other medications prescribed in addition to the antibiotics generally are taken for a longer period of time.

Acid blockers

Acid blockers — also called histamine (H-2) blockers — help relieve ulcer pain and encourage healing by reducing the amount of hydrochloric acid that's naturally released into your digestive tract. Normally, this acid doesn't damage your stomach and duodenum because of a protective layer of mucus coating the inside of your stomach and intestines. But if a defect or opening develops in the mucous layer, acid seeps into the defect and produces an ulcer.

Other factors, including regular use of nicotine and NSAIDs, increase the risk of a defect in the digestive lining turning into an ulcer.

Acid blockers do not kill *H. pylori*. They work by keeping histamine, a chemical that works with your immune system, from reaching histamine receptors. The receptors signal acid-secreting cells in your stomach to release hydrochloric acid. By blocking histamine, the acid blockers lower acid levels.

Available by prescription or over the counter, acid blockers include the medications cimetidine (Tagamet), famotidine (Pepcid), nizatidine (Axid) and ranitidine (Zantac). For treatment of ulcers, prescription acid blockers are more effective because they're stronger than the over-the-counter products.

Antacids

Your doctor may include an antacid in your drug regimen. The antacid may be taken in addition to an acid blocker or in place of one. Instead of reducing acid secretion, antacids neutralize existing stomach acid and provide pain relief.

Proton pump inhibitors

A more effective way to reduce stomach acid is by taking proton pump inhibitors (PPIs) rather than acid blockers. These medications shut down the action of tiny pumps at work within acid-secreting cells. Proton pump inhibitors also help kill *H. pylori* bacteria.

PPIs include the prescription medications dexlansoprazole (Dexilant), esomeprazole (Nexium), lansoprazole (Prevacid), omeprazole (Prilosec), omeprazole-sodium bicarbonate (Zegerid), pantoprazole (Protonix) and rabeprazole (Aciphex), and the over-the-counter medications omeprazole (Prilosec OTC) and lansoprazole (Prevacid 24HR). PPIs cost almost twice as much as acid blockers. Uncommon side effects include stomach pain, diarrhea, constipation and headache.

Cytoprotective agents

Cytoprotective agents help protect your body's cells, including tissues lining the stomach and small intestine, from dangerous chemicals and other factors.

They include the prescription medications sucralfate (Carafate) and misoprostol (Cytotec). Sucralfate may cause constipation. Misoprostol may cause diarrhea and bleeding. Misoprostol shouldn't be taken by women who are pregnant or planning to become pregnant because it can cause miscarriage.

Another cytoprotective agent is bismuth subsalicylate (Pepto-Bismol). In addition to its protective qualities, this agent appears to help kill *H. pylori*.

Self-care promotes healing

Before the discovery of *H. pylori*, people with ulcers were often placed on restricted diets and told to reduce the stress in their lives. Now that food and stress have been eliminated as causes of ulcers, these factors no longer apply.

However, while an ulcer is healing, it's still advisable to watch what you eat and to control stress. Eating acidic or spicy foods may increase ulcer pain.

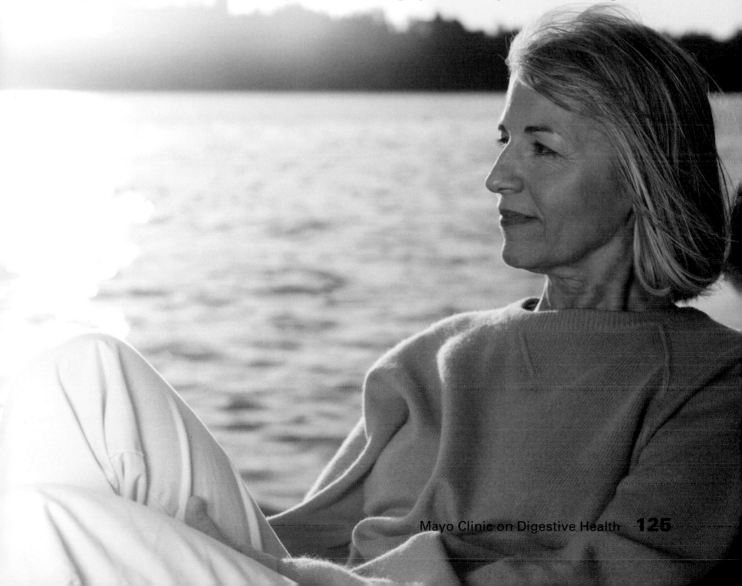

Periods of stress slow digestion, allowing food and digestive juices to remain in your stomach and intestines for longer periods of time. Your doctor may suggest taking the following tips:

- Don't smoke — smoking may delay ulcer healing
- Avoid alcohol
- Take acetaminophen (Tylenol, others) for pain relief

Nonulcer dyspepsia

Sometimes, people will see their doctors for what they think are the signs and symptoms of an ulcer. Although they may have gnawing upper abdominal pain, diagnostic tests don't reveal a digestive problem — all test results come back normal.

Many of these people have a condition known as nonulcer dyspepsia (dis-PEP-see-uh), or functional dyspepsia. It's a condition that brings the discomfort of an ulcer without an ulcer.

Nonulcer dyspepsia is common and can be long lasting. Unfortunately, it appears to occur for no apparent reason. Its most common symptom is pain, or an uncomfortable feeling, in your upper abdomen. Other signs and symptoms may include gas, bloating, nausea or feeling full after eating only a moderate amount of food.

As with ulcers, the pain is often, but not always, relieved with food or antacids. It's possible to control the condition with changes to your diet and lifestyle, but medications are sometimes helpful for managing the symptoms.

Plenty of theories, little proof

Although the cause (or causes) of nonulcer dyspepsia is largely unknown, it's possible that the pain stems from an irritation to your stomach lining. Researchers have considered other theories as well.

Presence of *H. pylori* bacteria
Your symptoms may represent an early case of *H. pylori* infection, despite the fact that no ulcer has developed.

Reaction to drugs and supplements
Pain relievers such as aspirin and other NSAIDs are known to cause ulcers and gastritis. It's possible these medications can irritate your digestive system without damaging your stomach or intestines. This may be true for other drugs

and supplements, including antibiotics, steroids, minerals and herbs.

Overproduction of stomach acid
Acid-secreting cells in your stomach may produce higher than normal amounts of digestive acid. The over-supply may irritate digestive tissues.

Stomach disorder
For unknown reasons, your stomach may not be functioning or emptying normally. This sometimes happens after certain viral infections.

Acid sensitivity
Tissues lining the stomach and duodenum may be overly sensitive to normal acid levels and become easily irritated.

Food sensitivity
Your stomach or intestines may be overly sensitive to certain kinds of food or food ingredients. Often, but not always, these include certain spices, citrus fruits or vegetables that contain moderate to high levels of acid. Some people find that drinking coffee seems to make the symptoms worse.

Overreaction to normal stimuli
Nerve signals between your stomach and brain may be faulty, resulting in an exaggerated response to the normal changes taking place during digestion, such as how your stomach stretches and expands as it fills with food. This overreaction is known as visceral hypersensitivity.

Stress
Pain may be your body's way of responding to periods of stress.

Psychological disorder
Depression, anxiety or another factor affecting your emotional health may have a role in causing your symptoms, for example, increasing your awareness and sensitivity to pain and discomfort.

Lifestyle changes are often the first steps

The symptoms of nonulcer dyspepsia are usually mild. Often the condition is treated by examining and changing your daily routines. This may include avoiding certain foods that seem to worsen symptoms, controlling stress, and changing or limiting daily medications or supplements. Some people find that having smaller but more frequent meals and eating low-fat foods also improves their symptoms.

If these practices don't help you, your doctor may recommend drug therapy. Many of the medications used to treat ulcers are recommended for nonulcer dyspepsia. At times, antibiotics are prescribed — some people with nonulcer dyspepsia test positive for *H. pylori*. Eradicating *H. pylori*, however, may not improve your symptoms. Other therapies that may be helpful include:

Pain relievers

Drugs that block pain or its perception may help desensitize nerves in your digestive system. Antidepressants often work well for irritable bowel syndrome, which some researchers believe may be associated with nonulcer dyspepsia. However, further study is needed to determine the value of antidepressant therapy.

Antispasmodic drugs

These drugs, including the prescription medications dicyclomine (Bentyl) and hyoscyamine (Levsin), help relax muscles in your digestive tract, but haven't shown much promise in treating nonulcer dyspepsia.

Behavior therapy

If your condition may be related to stress or a psychological disorder, you may see a psychiatrist, psychologist or nurse counselor. These health care professionals can help you control stress or deal with intense emotions that may be contributing to your symptoms.

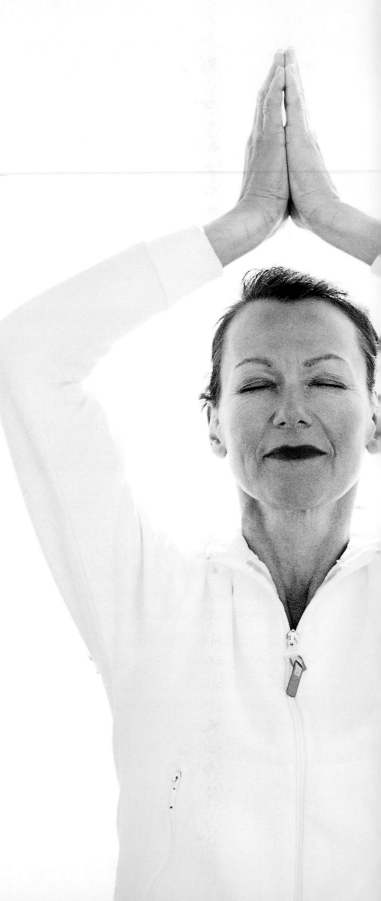

Chapter 7

Irritable bowel syndrome

You're out with friends, and you've just finished a delicious meal when the familiar rumblings in your stomach begin. You excuse yourself and head for home, where you spend the next hour dealing with cramps and diarrhea. On other occasions, you may battle uncomfortable constipation. Either way, your quality of life suffers.

Irritable bowel syndrome (IBS) is a common problem that affects about 1 in 5 adults in the United States, most commonly women. IBS is sometimes called spastic colon because for years spasms of the intestinal walls were thought to cause its symptoms. The walls of your intestines are lined with layers of muscle that contract and relax, helping to move food through your digestive tract (peristalsis, see also page 17).

Normally, the muscles contract and relax in coordinated rhythm. With IBS, the muscles may function abnormally. They may contract for a longer amount of time, and with greater force than normal, causing pain. Food is forced through the intestines more quickly, producing gas, bloating and diarrhea.

Key signs and symptoms

- Abdominal pain or discomfort
- Bloating or gas
- Diarrhea
- Constipation
- Mucus in stool

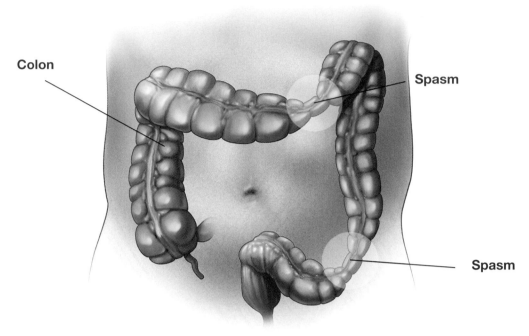

Colon

Spasm

Spasm

The highlighted areas represent severe muscle spasms that may occur in the large intestine (colon) causing pain. Spasms associated with irritable bowel syndrome can occur in one or more locations.

Sometimes, the opposite may occur. Contractions may be weak and the passage of food slows down, leading to hard, dry stools and constipation.

IBS is a disorder affecting the large intestine (colon). It's not life-threatening. If you have a mild form, the condition may be only a minor inconvenience — and most people have mild symptoms. Some people have moderate symptoms that are intermittent but can be disabling. At the other end of the spectrum, for the small fraction of people who have severe symptoms, the pain can seem unbearable.

A functional disorder

IBS is often referred to as a functional disorder, meaning that your intestines look normal, but they function abnormally. No one knows for certain what causes the dysfunction. Some researchers believe that the condition is related to nerves that control sensation. These nerves may be more sensitive than normal, causing you to react strongly to certain foods, physical activity, or the presence of air or gas in your intestines.

Something that might not bother most people, such as a little gas, may cause pain or bloating if you have IBS.

Researchers also feel that stress and other psychological factors contribute to IBS. Many people find that their symptoms are more severe or frequent during stressful events, such as changes in daily routine, having family troubles or attending social gatherings.

For years, doctors attributed IBS to stress alone. But studies suggest both a functional (physiological) and an emotional (psychological) basis. Some people with IBS have a history of physical, sexual or emotional abuse, which may contribute to the symptoms.

Because women are twice as likely as men to have IBS, researchers have speculated that hormonal changes may play a role. IBS may also result from another illness. Some people first experience IBS after an acute episode of diarrhea (postinfectious IBS).

IBS is not related to inflammatory bowel diseases such as Crohn's disease or ulcerative colitis. IBS also doesn't cause cancer or make you more likely to have cancer. IBS does run in families, and researchers are investigating the genetic component of the condition.

Ruling out other conditions

There are no tests that can confirm, without a doubt, that you have IBS. Typically, the disorder is diagnosed after other conditions that produce similar symptoms have been ruled out. In some but not all individuals suspected of having IBS, diagnostic tests may include blood, stool and urine tests, X-rays, colonoscopy, and transit studies. (See Chapter 4 for more about these tests.)

Your doctor also may ask about your emotional health. Are you undergoing periods of stress? How well do you cope with stress? Do you often feel depressed or anxious?

Before IBS is diagnosed, certain signs and symptoms — known as Rome criteria — must be present. The most important is abdominal pain or discomfort that has occurred at least three days a month over the previous three months. The pain must be accompanied by at least two or more of the following to support a diagnosis of IBS:

• Bowel movements that provide temporary relief from the pain or discomfort

- A change in how frequently you have bowel movements accompanies the onset of signs and symptoms — it can be more frequent or less frequent
- A change in the consistency of your stool accompanies the onset of signs and symptoms — it can be softer or firmer

Management with diet and exercise

Because there's no cure for IBS, treatment focus is on managing signs and symptoms. This will allow you to continue participating in normal activities and enjoying life more fully. Your success will depend on how well you achieve the following goals:

- Identify factors that trigger your signs and symptoms
- Develop strategies to minimize your signs and symptoms

A healthy diet and regular exercise are good starting points for managing IBS. They help keep your digestive system functioning smoothly. Keep in mind, however, that your body may not respond immediately to the changes you make. Instead, look for signs of gradual improvement. Your goal is to find long-term, not temporary, solutions.

Eat low-fat foods

Fat may stimulate the abnormal muscle contractions in your colon, only aggravating IBS symptoms. You don't need to avoid all fat in your diet, but if fat seems to worsen pain and diarrhea, try limiting the amount you eat.

The best way to reduce fat in your diet is to eat more plant-based foods. Plant foods — fruits, vegetables and foods made from whole grains — are naturally low in fat and contain many beneficial vitamins, minerals and cancer-preventing compounds (phytochemicals), as well as fiber.

Experiment with fiber

For people with IBS, dietary fiber can be either good or bad. High-fiber foods soften stool and speed its passage through your colon, reducing constipation. But for some people, increased fiber worsens diarrhea, gas and pain. It may be that these individuals are more sensitive to gases produced in the colon from the fermentation of fiber.

Is it IBS or is it a food intolerance?

If your cramping and bloating occur mainly after eating dairy products or sugar-free gum or candies, your problem may not be irritable bowel syndrome but another condition.

People with lactose intolerance have difficulty digesting the sugar (lactose) in dairy products because their bodies don't produce enough of the enzyme lactase — a substance normally found in the small intestine. Lactase breaks down lactose so that it can be absorbed into your body. When lactose isn't absorbed, it travels to the colon where fermentation takes place — normal bacteria convert the lactose to gas and fluid, causing cramping and diarrhea.

Fructose is a natural sugar, like glucose, that does not require enzymes in order for you to digest it. But unlike glucose, your small intestine can absorb only so much fructose in one day. If you ingest too much fructose, the excess passes into your colon where normal bacteria convert it to gas and fluid, causing cramping and diarrhea. Fructose is found in most fruits, especially apricots, cherries, peaches, pears, plums and prunes, as well as fruit juices, honey and processed foods with added fructose-containing corn syrup. This includes most nondiet soft drinks.

The artificial sweetener sorbitol (as well as other compounds) found in some gums and candies also can produce symptoms similar to those of IBS. If cramping and abdominal pain typically occur after chewing sugar-free gum or eating sugar-free candy, your problem could be an intolerance to sorbitol.

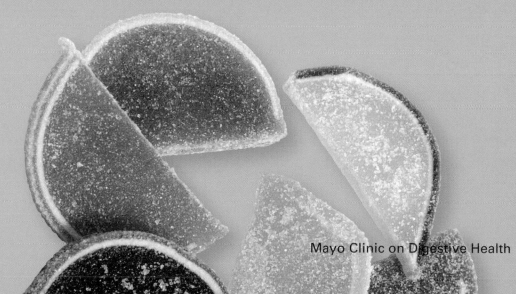

The best approach is to increase the amount of fiber in your diet gradually over a period of weeks and gauge your body's response. If you take this action and continue to experience pain or diarrhea, you may need to pursue a different path. Consult with a dietitian about a low-fat diet that also includes reduced amounts of dietary fiber.

For more information on eating healthy and adjusting the amount of fiber in your diet, see pages 31-35.

Drink plenty of liquids

Include plenty of beverages in your diet to help relieve constipation and to replenish body fluids that are absorbed by fiber during the digestive process. Make it your goal each day to drink at least eight glasses of fluid. Water is your best choice.

Beverages containing caffeine or alcohol cause you to urinate more — essentially helping to reduce rather than increase body fluids. They may also worsen diarrhea by stimulating or irritating your intestines. Avoid carbonated beverages because they can produce gas, which may add to the discomfort and bloating you already feel from IBS.

Avoid problem foods

Many people with IBS notice improvements in signs and symptoms simply by excluding certain foods or beverages from their diets. Common culprits include fatty foods, beans and other legumes, alcohol and caffeine. For more on gas-producing foods, see page 57.

Eat at regular times

Don't skip meals. And try to eat at about the same times each day. Regularly scheduled meals, including breakfast, help regulate your bowel function and lessen symptoms of constipation and diarrhea. That's because digestion involves stimulating the muscles in your gastrointestinal tract to contract and relax — the process necessary to move stool through your colon and into your rectum.

Some people find that eating frequent, smaller meals agrees with them better than does eating three large meals a day. For others, especially people bothered by constipation, the opposite may be true. To stimulate muscle contractions and the passage of stool, they need to eat medium-sized to large meals. Either option is acceptable if it helps you manage your symptoms.

Get active

Physical activity helps reduce feelings of stress. It also stimulates the regular rhythmic muscle contractions of your intestines, helping them to function normally. Physical activity can relieve constipation and also may alleviate symptoms of diarrhea. Exercise can also improve depression and make you feel better about yourself.

Aim for 30 to 60 minutes of moderate physical activity on most days of the week. If you've been inactive, begin slowly, and then gradually increase the time you exercise. For information on the benefits of exercise and setting up a fitness program, see "Get regular exercise" on pages 43-46.

Other helpful hints

These steps also may help relieve some signs and symptoms of IBS:

- Soak in a warm bath or lie down with a hot-water bottle or heating pad on your abdomen to decrease abdominal pain. Be careful not to burn your skin or to fall asleep.
- Wear comfortable, loosefitting clothing so as not to put pressure on your abdomen.

- Go to the bathroom as soon as you feel the urge, but don't hurry yourself. Allow adequate time for a bowel movement without straining.
- Eat breakfast as soon as you get up in the morning.

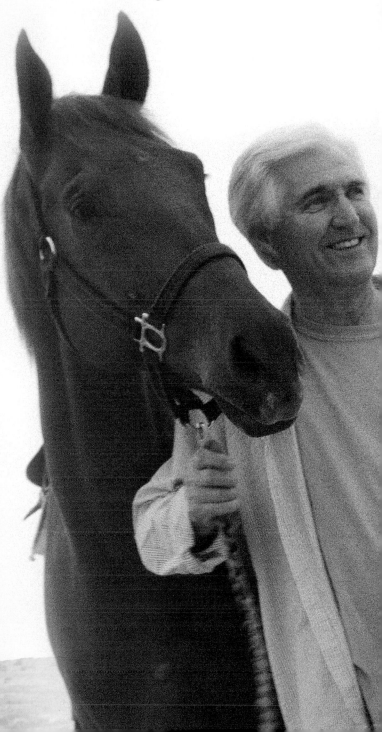

Taking a breather

Here's an exercise to help you practice deep, relaxed breathing. Rehearse throughout the day until you can automatically apply the exercise when you feel stressed:

1. Sit comfortably with your feet flat on the floor.
2. Loosen tight clothing around your abdomen and waist.
3. Place your hands on your lap or at your sides.
4. Close your eyes if it helps you to relax.
5. Breathe in slowly through your nose while counting to four. Allow your abdomen to expand as you breathe in.
6. Pause for a second and then exhale at a normal rate through your mouth.
7. Repeat until you feel more relaxed.

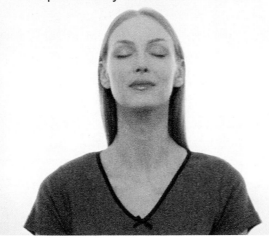

Learning to manage stress

Anyone can experience digestive upset from worry, anxiety or other stressful emotions. But if you have IBS, stress-related symptoms such as abdominal pain and diarrhea tend to occur more frequently and severely. A vicious cycle may develop — your signs and symptoms increase the level of stress, more stress causes your signs and symptoms to worsen, and so on.

An important strategy in controlling IBS is learning how to relax. There are many methods of relaxation. Some people relax while listening to or performing music, or surrounding themselves with soothing aromas (aromatherapy). Others benefit from massage, yoga or meditation.

Studies show that hypnosis also may reduce abdominal pain and bloating. A trained professional instructs you on how to enter a relaxed (hypnotic) state and guides you through an imagery session during which you imagine your bowel muscles smooth, calm and still.

To help you get started in managing stress, here are two simple techniques for whenever you feel a need to relax.

Deep breathing

Stress typically causes rapid, shallow breathing from your chest. Deep, slow, relaxed breathing comes from your diaphragm, the muscle separating your chest from your abdomen. More relaxed breathing means your abdomen, not your chest, moves with each breath.

The sidebar "Taking a breather" shows you how to breathe from your diaphragm. You can use deep breathing as your only means of relaxation or as a warm-up and cool-down method for other techniques.

Progressive muscle relaxation

This technique involves relaxing various muscle groups, one at a time. First, increase the tension level in one muscle group, such as a leg or an arm, by tightening the muscles. Then relax the muscles. Focus on slowly letting the tension subside. Then, move on to the next muscle group in similar fashion.

Over-the-counter medications

Nonprescription medications may help relieve discomfort at the same time that you're taking steps to change or improve your lifestyle. Most pharmacies, drugstores and grocery stores will carry these over-the-counter products. Which products you use will depend on your signs and symptoms.

Anti-diarrheals

Relieving symptoms of diarrhea is often one of your most important concerns for managing IBS. Loperamide (Imodium) slows the rate at which food leaves your intestines and increases water and sodium absorption, both of which help solidify stool. Other anti-diarrheals, such as bismuth subsalicylate (Pepto-Bismol), also may ease the urgency of a bowel movement.

You need to be careful, however, not to use anti-diarrheal medications too often or for too long. Talk with your doctor about safe and effective use. One approach would be to take an anti-diarrheal after each loose bowel movement. That way, the amount of treatment can match the severity of the diarrhea. Some people take an anti-diarrheal before they go out to eat, to serve as a safety net and to avoid embarrassment.

You might also experiment with peppermint tea (tea that contains peppermint oil). There's some evidence it helps relieve diarrhea or gas accompanied by bloating. However, peppermint can also aggravate heartburn.

Fiber supplements and laxatives

To help relieve signs and symptoms of constipation, try using a natural fiber supplement such as Metamucil or Citrucel. (For more on fiber, see pages 31-35.) Start by using a small amount, such as a teaspoon of supplement mixed in a glass of water or juice, and slowly increase your daily dose every one to two weeks. When taken regularly as directed, fiber supplements are generally safe and effective.

Because they're so absorbent, take fiber supplements with plenty of water. Otherwise, they can become constipating — the opposite of what you want. If these measures don't help, ask your doctor about using a laxative. There are several types.

Stool softeners
Sold over-the-counter under several brand names, including Colace and Surfak, stool softeners are the most gentle laxatives.

Avoid taking mineral oil to help soften your stools and relieve constipation.

Mineral oil can block the absorption of key vitamins. Never take mineral oil before lying down, as it could enter your lungs and cause pneumonia.

Saline laxatives
Saline laxatives are relatively safe to use and include Phillips' Milk of Magnesia and Miralax. They work by increasing water content in your stool.

Stimulant laxatives
The most powerful type of laxative, stimulant laxatives should be considered when other measures fail to induce a bowel movement. But first, discuss their use with your doctor. Over-the-counter brand names include Dulcolax, Ex-Lax and Senokot.

Avoid the long-term, unsupervised use of these products. Talk with your doctor about the best approach for using any over-the-counter laxatives.

Treating severe symptoms

If signs and symptoms of IBS are moderate to severe, you may need more help than what lifestyle changes or over-the-counter medications can offer.

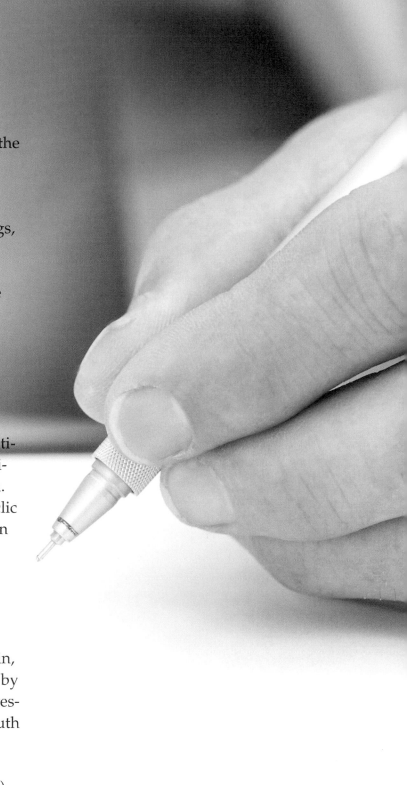

Prescription medications

Depending on signs and symptoms, your doctor may recommend one of the following prescription medications.

Smooth-muscle relaxants
Anticholinergic (antispasmodic) drugs, such as hyoscyamine (Levsin) and dicyclomine (Bentyl), may help relax intestinal muscles and relieve muscle spasms. The medications have many side effects, including urinary retention, accelerated heart rate, blurred vision and dry mouth.

Antidepressants
In addition to treating depression, antidepressants may help relieve abdominal pain and diarrhea or constipation. Your doctor may recommend a tricyclic antidepressant or a selective serotonin reuptake inhibitor (SSRI).

The tricyclic agents amitriptyline, doxepin, imipramine (Tofranil) and nortriptyline (Pamelor) are most frequently prescribed for abdominal pain, especially if the pain is accompanied by attacks of diarrhea. Tricyclic antidepressants may cause drowsiness, dry mouth and constipation.

The SSRIs fluoxetine (Prozac, Sarafem) and paroxetine (Paxil) are recommended for abdominal pain. However, in some people SSRIs can cause nausea, cramping and diarrhea.

Antidepressants must be taken regularly to be effective. Because of this, these medications generally are prescribed only if you have chronic or recurring symptoms.

Lubiprostone

Lubiprostone (Amitiza) is a prescription laxative that stimulates the secretion of intestinal fluids, which helps move food through the intestines. Headache and nausea may occur as side effects.

Counseling

This is an important aspect of treatment if your condition is related to stress. A health care professional who specializes in behavioral medicine, such as a psychiatrist or psychologist, can help you reduce stress and anxiety by examining your responses to life events, and then helping you modify those responses. You learn to identify stressful situations that cause bowel reactions and develop strategies for controlling stress. For most people, counseling combined with medication works better than does medication alone.

Chapter 8

Crohn's disease and ulcerative colitis

Crohn's disease and ulcerative colitis are the two most common forms of inflammatory bowel disease (IBD), an umbrella term for inflammatory conditions, many of them chronic, that can damage the digestive tract.

Key signs and symptoms

- Diarrhea
- Abdominal pain and cramping
- Blood in stool
- Fatigue
- Reduced appetite
- Weight loss
- Fever

A primary concern for many people with inflammatory bowel disease is managing chronic diarrhea or rectal bleeding. Some people experience just a couple of episodes of diarrhea daily, while others may have more than a half-dozen. Among people with severe forms of IBD, daily life revolves around constant fear of a sudden, urgent bowel movement and making sure that a bathroom is close by.

There is no cure for Crohn's disease, named after Burrill Crohn, M.D., who, along with his colleagues, described the disease in 1932. There is only one cure for ulcerative colitis, which is surgical removal of the colon and rectum.

But there is also good news for people with IBD. Although these diseases often can't be cured, their signs and symptoms can be treated. Several therapies can dramatically improve your condition, and possibly even produce a long-term remission — a period of time when the signs and symptoms of disease diminish.

Similar but different

Crohn's disease and ulcerative colitis share many of the same signs and symptoms. They can behave so similarly, in fact, that one condition is sometimes mistaken for the other. Both conditions inflame the inner lining of the digestive tract. Both can take an unpredictable course, such as severe flare-ups, sometimes long term, followed by extended periods of remission. And both may require a complex plan of drug therapy, often using nearly identical medications.

Despite these similarities, the two conditions exhibit several key differences. Crohn's disease can occur anywhere in your digestive tract, from your mouth to your anus, although its most common location is the small intestine. It can develop in different locations si-

multaneously in patches. Inflammation generally settles into the deepest layers of tissue in the affected areas.

Ulcerative colitis is limited to the colon and rectum. The inflammation often begins in the rectum and then spreads in long, continuous stretches into the colon. The disease differs from Crohn's in that only the thin lining of the inner surface is inflamed and typically the deeper tissues aren't affected.

Though Crohn's disease and ulcerative colitis can occur at any age, the diseases tend to affect people within two different ranges in age: between ages 15 and 35 and between ages 50 and 80. Men and women are equally susceptible. Whites have the highest risk of IBD, but the disease occurs in many different ethnic groups. In particular, Jewish people of European descent are five times as likely to have inflammatory bowel disease as are other whites.

Crohn's disease and ulcerative colitis together affect over 1 million Americans, with each condition accounting for roughly half that number. Some estimates are twice as high. Wide variation in the estimates of prevalence is partly due to the diseases being difficult to diagnose and many people being unaware they have a condition.

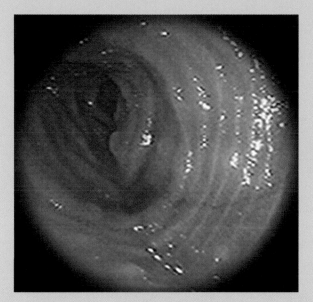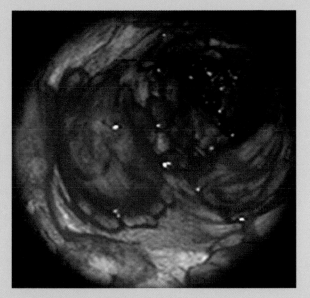

The endoscopic image at left is a healthy interior of the small intestine with even coloration and well-spaced, circular folds. The image at right shows the small intestine with a "rake-type" pattern of inflammation characteristic of Crohn's disease. Mucous membrane forms bumpy nodules along the margins.

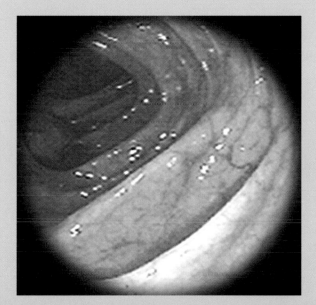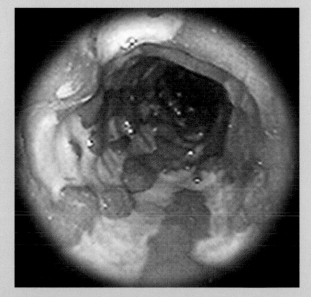

The endoscopic image at left shows typical folding and tissue coloration in the transverse colon. The image at right reveals ulcerative colitis extending in long, continuous stretches into the colon. The inflammation develops only in the thin lining of the inner surface.

In search of a cause

Although researchers haven't unlocked the mysteries behind the causes of Crohn's disease and ulcerative colitis, there's a general consensus as to what doesn't cause them. Contrary to past belief, researchers no longer believe that stress and troubled emotional health are the culprits — although they may aggravate symptoms.

Nor do researchers think the diseases are due to sensitivities to certain foods or passed on by infection from one person to another.

As for factors that may trigger IBD, there are only theories for the moment:

Immune system
One theory holds that the diseases are linked to infection from an unknown virus or bacteria. Inflammation typically is a result of your body's immune system trying to fight off the invaders. It's a fact that drugs used to suppress the immune system are also proving to be remarkably effective at controlling the signs and symptoms of IBD in many people. It also is possible that the inflammation may stem directly from a viral or bacterial infection.

Still another possibility is that your immune system is mistaking beneficial bacteria that normally live in your intestinal tract as a threat to your body and attacking them.

Heredity
Fifteen to 30 percent of people with Crohn's disease or ulcerative colitis have an immediate family member — parent, brother, sister or child — with IBD. The multiple genetic factors that may make a person susceptible to inflammatory conditions are the subject of intensive research.

Researchers have learned that mutations in one particular gene occur frequently in people with Crohn's disease. This gene, known as NOD2, plays a role in stimulating your immune system to fight invading bacteria.

Environment
Both diseases are more prevalent in developed nations and in cities. This has led some experts to speculate that environmental factors, such as diet, may play a role. Another theory is that people living in cleaner environments may in essence be victims of good hygiene and public health measures. As a result, they become more vulnerable to infections later in life, causing their immune systems to overreact.

Signs and symptoms

Both Crohn's disease and ulcerative colitis produce a variety of signs and symptoms, which may appear suddenly or develop gradually.

Crohn's disease

One or more of the following signs and symptoms may occur in mild to severe forms with Crohn's disease:

Diarrhea

Your intestines respond to inflammation in the same way they respond to infection. As part of the process, your cells may secrete extra amounts of salt and water, overwhelming the capacity of your intestinal tract to absorb fluid. At the same time, muscles in your intestinal walls may contract more frequently. The result is diarrhea.

Cramping and vomiting

Persistent inflammation in the intestinal tract can cause scar tissue to form, which contributes to the swelling and thickening of intestinal walls. Intestinal channels may narrow, blocking the passage of food waste. Cramping and vomiting can result.

Is Crohn's disease mild, moderate or severe?

✓ **Mild Crohn's disease**
- Four or fewer diarrheal bowel movements daily
- Minimal abdominal pain or no pain at all
- Healthy weight
- Few, if any, complications
- Normal temperature, pulse and red blood cell count

✓ **Moderate Crohn's disease**
- Four to six diarrheal bowel movements daily
- Moderate abdominal pain
- Additional complications

✓ **Severe Crohn's disease**
- Six or more diarrheal bowel movements daily
- Severe abdominal pain
- Underweight
- Additional complications
- Fever, rapid pulse, low red blood cell count, high white blood cell count

Bleeding

As food waste touches or rubs against inflamed tissue on its passage through your intestinal tract, the tissue may bleed. Inflamed tissue may also bleed without food waste. The blood expelled with your stool may appear bright red in the toilet bowl or dark in color when mixed in with stool.

Weight loss and fatigue

Due to inflammation in your small intestine, you may be unable to absorb sufficient amounts of nutrients to maintain weight and energy level. So you lose pounds and tire easily. Excessive blood loss also can produce fatigue. Malabsorption of nutrients may be the reason why children with Crohn's disease tend to have stunted growth.

Ulcers

Chronic inflammation can produce open sores (ulcers) in your intestinal tract. Some people develop a string of disconnected ulcers throughout the tract, even in the mouth, esophagus or anus. Typically, Crohn's-related ulcers develop in the lower small intestine (terminal ileum), colon and rectum.

Fistulas

Ulcers may burrow completely through the intestinal wall and create a fistula — an abnormal, tubular connection between organs or to the surface of the skin. Often, fistulas connect one loop of the small intestine to another. When a fistula develops between the small intestine and colon, food particles take a shortcut through the opening and arrive in the colon before their nutrients have been fully absorbed.

Sometimes, a fistula can develop into a pocket of infection (abscess), which can become life-threatening. Treatment may involve medication or surgery.

Other complications

Crohn's disease can cause additional problems, including:

- Inflammation, swelling, stiffness and pain in your joints
- Skin rashes or sores
- Anal skin tags, which mimic hemorrhoids
- Inflammation of your eyes
- Kidney stones
- Gallstones
- Colon cancer

It's uncertain what causes these complications. Some researchers believe they're all linked to an immune system response in parts of your body other than the digestive tract. When the disease is treated, some signs and symptoms will disappear.

Ulcerative colitis

Similar to Crohn's disease, ulcerative colitis can cause diarrhea, bleeding, cramping and abdominal pain, as well as complications such as skin rash, arthritis and eye inflammation. However, ulcerative colitis is more often associated with liver disease than with kidney stones, gallstones or anal skin tags. With ulcerative colitis, your stool often is mixed with blood, in addition to mucus or pus.

Toxic megacolon is a serious complication of ulcerative colitis that can occur in some individuals. The inflamed colon becomes immobilized and distended, unable to expel stool and gas. Signs and symptoms include abdominal pain and swelling, fever, and weakness. You may also become groggy or disoriented. Left untreated, the colon may rupture and bacteria from the colon infects the abdominal cavity, a condition called peritonitis that can be fatal. A ruptured colon requires emergency surgery.

Long-term ulcerative colitis involving a substantial portion of the colon and rectum increases your risk of colorectal cancer. Regular screenings with colonoscopy is recommended after eight to 10 years of the disease.

Is ulcerative colitis mild, moderate or severe?

✓ **Mild ulcerative colitis**
- Four or fewer diarrheal bowel movements daily
- Occasional blood in stool
- Few, if any, complications
- Normal temperature, pulse and red blood cell count

✓ **Moderate ulcerative colitis**
- Four to six diarrheal bowel movements daily
- Blood in stool fairly regularly
- Additional complications

✓ **Severe ulcerative colitis**
- Six or more diarrheal bowel movements daily
- Frequent blood in stool
- Tender abdomen
- Additional complications
- Fever, rapid pulse, low red blood cell count, high white blood cell count

Diagnosing IBD

There's no single test that your doctor can rely on to definitively diagnose Crohn's disease or ulcerative colitis. Like many other digestive conditions, typical signs and symptoms may be associated with any number of other diseases. Inflammatory bowel disease is most often diagnosed following a series of tests that are able to rule out other probable causes.

Diagnostic tests that may help confirm Crohn's disease or ulcerative colitis include the following:

Blood tests

Blood tests identify the levels of certain substances in your bloodstream. Some tests can check the level of C-reactive protein (CRP), which is produced in your liver, or for abnormal erythrocyte sedimentation rates (ESR). Both tests can indicate the presence of inflammation somewhere in your body, although neither can pinpoint its exact location.

Two other tests — perinuclear anti-neutrophilic cytoplasmic antibody (pANCA) and anti-saccharomyces cerevisiae antibody (ASCA) — can occasionally help diagnose the presence of inflammatory bowel disease.

X-rays

X-ray images of your small and large intestines may detect ulcers, swelling or complications such as the formation of a stricture or fistula. For more on this procedure, see pages 78-81.

Colonoscopy

This endoscopic exam is the best procedure for diagnosing Crohn's disease or ulcerative colitis. The doctor uses a flexible tube equipped with a camera to relay images of your digestive tract to an external monitor. For more on this procedure, see pages 86-88.

If the inner walls of your intestines are inflamed, they will bleed easily when gently touched by the endoscope. Areas of inflammation interspersed with areas of normal tissue suggests Crohn's disease. A continuous area of inflammation suggests ulcerative colitis.

During the test, your doctor may also retrieve tissue samples (biopsy) that will be examined under a microscope. Granulomas in the samples may confirm Crohn's disease, but often they're not present. Granulomas are small groupings of inflammatory cells that typically attempt to surround and destroy bacteria and other foreign bodies. Granulomas don't usually occur with ulcerative colitis.

Helpful medications

Medications can't cure inflammatory bowel disease (IBD), but they can effectively reduce the signs and symptoms in most people and improve quality of life. The primary goal of drug therapy is reducing inflammation in the intestinal tract, because that's what triggers most of the problems.

Doctors rely on several categories of drugs that help control inflammation in different ways. Some of these drugs may work well for some people but not for others. So it may take time to discover what works best for you.

Anti-inflammatory drugs

Anti-inflammatory drugs are often a first step in treating IBD. These drugs inhibit the release of enzymes that trigger the inflammatory process.

Sulfasalazine

This medication has been commonly prescribed for mild to moderate ulcerative colitis — less often for Crohn's disease — since the 1940s. Sulfasalazine (Azulfidine) often effectively reduces signs and symptoms of both diseases and can help prevent a relapse of ulcerative colitis. The medication is relatively inexpensive. Side effects may include loss of appetite, nausea, vomiting, skin rash and headache.

Mesalamine, balsalazide and olsalazine

More recently, doctors have turned to mesalamine (Asacol, Rowasa, others), balsalazide (Colazal) and olsalazine (Dipentum). These drugs work in similar fashion to sulfasalazine, but they typically produce fewer side effects. You can take the medications in tablet form or use them rectally as enemas or suppositories. Your doctor may prescribe a combination of two different forms, such as an oral prescription and an enema or suppository.

Mesalamine enemas can relieve signs and symptoms of ulcerative colitis in the lower (sigmoid) colon and rectum. You administer the enema at night, while lying on your left side so that the medication bathes this section of your bowels. Treatment continues every night for four to eight weeks or until your intestinal lining has healed. The drawback of this therapy is that retaining the medication in your system can be difficult if your colon is very active. Suppositories may be used when the disease is limited to your rectum.

Corticosteroids

Steroids effectively reduce inflammation regardless of where the disease has developed, but they can cause numerous side effects, including weight gain, excessive facial hair, insomnia, irritability and hyperactivity. More-serious side effects include high blood pressure, diabetes, osteoporosis, cataracts, glaucoma and increased risk of infection. In children, prolonged use of steroids can stunt growth and development.

Corticosteroids are prescribed mainly for moderate to severe IBD that doesn't respond to other treatment. The drugs aren't intended for long-term use and are generally prescribed for three to four months. Commonly used steroids include prednisone, methylprednisolone and hydrocortisone. Slower acting steroids, such as budesonide (Entocort EC), are proving effective for mild to moderate Crohn's disease of the terminal ileum and first part of the colon.

Corticosteroids can be taken in tablet form or used rectally as a suppository, enema or foam. Rectal preparations are generally recommended for mild to moderate ulcerative colitis in the sigmoid colon or rectum. Intravenous steroids may be given if your condition is serious and requires hospitalization.

Immunosuppressants

Immunosuppressants reduce inflammation in a different way from anti-inflammatory drugs. They target your immune system, which may be causing the inflammation or contributing to it. One theory holds that your immune system overreacts to a viral or bacterial attack. To destroy the foreign agents, your immune system releases certain chemicals. Over time, these chemicals damage digestive tissues, causing inflammation. Immunosuppressive drugs relieve IBD by interfering with your immune system's ability to release the chemicals.

Azathioprine and mercaptopurine

These drugs are the most widely used immunosuppressants for treating inflammatory bowel disease. Exactly how the drugs work remains unclear, but it can take up to three months before they work optimally. Studies have found azathioprine (Azasan, Imuran) and mercaptopurine (Purinethol) are effective in reducing signs and symptoms of IBD and healing fistulas from Crohn's disease. They are also used long term to prevent the disease from reactivating.

Cyclosporine

This potent drug is often used if you don't respond well to other medications. Cyclosporine (Sandimmune) may improve the signs and symptoms of severe ulcerative colitis. The drug is effective within one to two weeks, and may be used to control symptoms until less toxic drugs start working.

Cyclosporine can produce significant side effects, including excessive hair growth, numbness of your hands and feet, seizures, high blood pressure, and liver and kidney damage.

Infliximab

Infliximab (Remicade) is an effective treatment for moderate to severe Crohn's disease as well as ulcerative colitis. The drug neutralizes a natural protein in your body called tumor necrosis factor (TNF) that causes inflammation. Infliximab finds TNF in your bloodstream before it triggers the inflammation in your intestinal tract. Infliximab is given as an intravenous (IV) infusion and once started, often continued as long-term therapy. Similar immunosuppressant drugs, adalimumab (Humira) and certolizumab pegol (Cimzia), are given as under-the-skin (subcutaneous) injections.

Methotrexate

A drug that's long been used to treat psoriasis and rheumatoid arthritis in addition to cancer, methotrexate is sometimes recommended for people with Crohn's disease who can't tolerate or don't respond well to other medications. Short-term side effects may include nausea. Long-term use of the drug may lead to scarring of the liver, but this is uncommon.

All immunosuppressive therapies require close monitoring by your doctor in order to reduce the risk of toxicity.

Blood tests are done regularly while you take immunosuppressants, and dosages may need to be adjusted depending on the results.

Antibiotics

Antibiotics generally aren't effective for ulcerative colitis, but for some people with Crohn's disease, this class of drugs can help heal fistulas and abscesses and possibly cause a remission of signs and symptoms. It's believed that antibiotics help reduce harmful intestinal bacteria and suppress the immune system, which may cause other side effects.

Metronidazole

This is one of the more commonly used antibiotics for Crohn's disease. Side effects of metronidazole (Flagyl), especially when used for more than two weeks, can include numbness and tingling in your hands and feet and, sometimes, pain and muscle weakness. Reversal of these signs and symptoms is slow, and they may never disappear. Less serious side effects include nausea, headache, yeast infection and loss of appetite. In addition, the drug may cause a metallic taste. Hard candy or chewing gum can help mask the taste. Consuming alcohol while taking metronidazole can lead to severe side effects.

Ciprofloxacin

An alternative to metronidazole is ciprofloxacin (Cipro). It improves signs and symptoms in some but not all people with Crohn's disease. Side effects include hypersensitivity to light, tendon rupture and, in children, possible stunting of growth.

Others

Tetracycline or the combination of sulfamethoxazole and trimethoprim (Bactrim, Septra) sometimes are used to treat Crohn's disease. Side effects can include numbness and tingling in your hands and feet. Long-term use is generally required to prevent relapse.

Nicotine gum and patches

In clinical trials, nicotine gum and skin patches — the products that smokers use to help them stop using tobacco products — appear to provide short-term relief from flare-ups of ulcerative colitis. A small, steady nicotine dose supplied by gum or patch eliminates signs and symptoms in some people. However, this treatment appears to be effective only for a short period of time, then signs and symptoms reappear.

How nicotine works to ease inflammation isn't clear. Researchers suspect it may protect the colon by thickening and increasing the mucous layer that covers intestinal lining where inflammation typically occurs. Nicotine may also reduce the actual inflammation.

Other medications

In addition to using drug therapy to control inflammation from Crohn's disease and ulcerative colitis, your doctor may also prescribe certain medications to help relieve other troublesome signs and symptoms. Depending on how severe these signs and symptoms are, your doctor may recommend one or more of the following drugs:

Anti-diarrheals
For mild to moderate diarrhea, a teaspoon of fiber supplement (Metamucil, Citrucel) mixed with water once or twice a day may reduce diarrhea. Fiber adds bulk to stool as it absorbs water.

For more severe diarrhea, loperamide (Imodium) or prescription narcotics can relax and slow the movement of your intestinal muscles. Narcotics, however, must be used with caution because they can produce side effects, including risk of toxic megacolon (see page 147).

Laxatives
The narrowing of intestinal passages due to swelling can occasionally lead to constipation. Laxatives can help prevent constipation, but ask your doctor before taking any laxative. Even popular over-the-counter brands can be too harsh on your digestive system.

Pain relievers
For mild pain, your doctor may recommend acetaminophen (Tylenol, others). Avoid nonsteroidal anti-inflammatory drugs (NSAIDs), such as aspirin, ibuprofen (Advil, Motrin, others), naproxen (Aleve) and ketoprofen. They may aggravate rather than reduce the signs and symptoms of IBD. For moderate to severe pain, a prescription drug may be more effective.

Iron supplements
Blood loss from intestinal bleeding can cause iron deficiency anemia. Iron supplements help restore adequate blood levels of iron and cure this type of anemia. The hormone erythropoietin is being tested for severe cases of anemia that don't respond to iron supplements alone. Erythropoietin works in your bone marrow to increase the production of red blood cells.

Vitamin B-12 injections
Vitamin B-12 is absorbed in the terminal ileum, a section of the small intestine commonly affected by Crohn's disease. If Crohn's is preventing the absorption of this vitamin, you may need B-12 shots once a month for the rest of your life. People who have a portion of the terminal ileum removed due to surgery (see pages 157-158) also require lifelong B-12 injections.

Living with IBD

Your experience with inflammatory bowel disease may include extended periods of remission when the condition is not as troublesome. But typically the signs and symptoms return, and you again face the discomfort and concern of living with IBD. In addition to the medication your doctor prescribes, the following steps can help you manage your signs and symptoms and lengthen the time between flare-ups.

Manage your diet

There's no firm evidence to suggest that the types of food you eat contribute to inflammatory bowel disease. However, it's true sometimes that certain foods and beverages appear to aggravate your signs and symptoms, especially during a flare-up in your condition.

It's also important to understand that what applies to someone else may not apply to you. Some people with IBD may need to restrict their diet all of the time, others only some of the time, and still others almost never.

If you suspect that a certain kind of food may make your condition worse, experiment with different foods and beverages to see if eliminating one or adding another helps you feel better. Do your experimenting carefully. Try these steps:

Limit dairy products
Some people with Crohn's disease and ulcerative colitis reduce diarrhea, pain and gas when they limit their consumption of dairy products. These people may be lactose intolerant (see pages 58-59). They aren't able to digest the lactose in dairy products because their bodies don't produce enough of the enzyme that breaks the substance down for absorption. If you find that dairy products seem to worsen your signs and symptoms, talk with a registered dietitian about designing a healthy, low-lactose diet.

Restrict fiber
High-fiber foods, such as fruits, vegetables and grains, are the foundation of a healthy diet. But for some people with inflammatory bowel disease, fiber can have a laxative effect, worsening diarrhea. Fiber can also increase gas. Experiment with high-fiber foods to see if you're able to tolerate some better than others. If fiber remains a problem, you may have to restrict fruits, vegetables and grains in your diet. A dietitian can help you replace the nutrients that these foods provide.

Reduce fat

People with severe Crohn's disease sometimes need to reduce the fat in their diets because their small intestine is no longer able to absorb fat. Instead, the fat passes through the digestive tract, causing or worsening diarrhea. Reducing fat in your diet generally isn't a problem, but if you're unable to maintain a healthy weight, talk with your doctor about increasing calories without increasing fat.

Ask about multivitamins

Because IBD can interfere with the normal absorption of nutrients, your doctor may also suggest taking a multivitamin that provides the Recommended Dietary Allowance (RDA) for essential vitamins and minerals. Supplements should be taken only under your doctor's supervision because they can interfere with medication or your body's ability to absorb nutrients.

Drink plenty of fluids

Beverages offset fluid loss from diarrhea. Drink at least eight 8-ounce glasses of fluid, preferably water, daily. Avoid beverages that contain caffeine or alcohol, which promote urination and fluid loss.

Reduce stress

Stress doesn't cause inflammatory bowel disease, but it may worsen your signs and symptoms and spark flare-ups. Many people with IBD report an increase in digestive problems when they're under moderate to severe stress.

Normal digestion changes due to stress. Your stomach empties more slowly and acid-secreting cells release more digestive juices. Stress also speeds or slows the passage of food through your intestines, although much is still unknown about why this happens.

Some forms of stress you can't avoid. But you can manage a lot of daily stress with exercise, adequate rest and taking time to relax, whether it's by listening to music or with meditation.

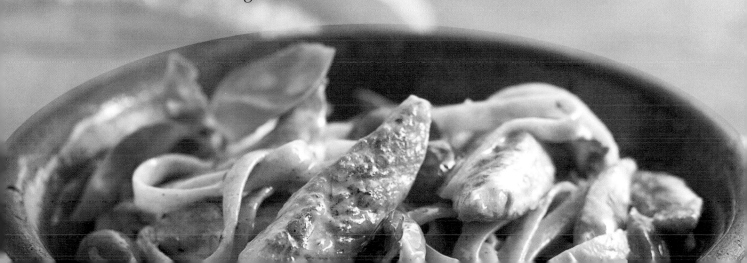

Crohn's, colitis and colon cancer

Both Crohn's disease and ulcerative colitis can increase your risk of colon cancer. If you've had inflammatory bowel disease of the colon for eight or more years, ask your doctor about screening for colon cancer every one to two years. The most effective test is colonoscopy (see pages 86-88).

For Crohn's disease of the colon, how long you've had the disease and the extent of the damage are key factors. The more time and the more of the colon involved, the greater your risk of colon cancer. Colon cancer, however, tends to be less common with Crohn's disease because, unlike ulcerative colitis, Crohn's disease usually doesn't affect the entire colon and the damaged portion has often been removed with surgery.

For ulcerative colitis, risk of colon cancer also depends on how long you've had the disease and how much of your colon is affected. You're at increased risk of colon cancer if you've had ulcerative colitis for eight to 10 years and if the disease involves more than just your rectum. The smaller the area of the colon that's diseased, generally the lower the risk of cancer.

Seek information and support

Beyond the physical manifestations, Crohn's disease and ulcerative colitis may also cause deep emotional scars. Chronic diarrhea may lead to embarrassing accidents. Some people become so humiliated socially that they isolate themselves, rarely leaving home. When they do go out, anxiety often makes their condition worse. Left untreated, these factors — isolation, humiliation, anxiety — can severely affect quality of life and lead to depression.

Many people with IBD find emotional support simply by learning more about their disease. They benefit from talking with medical professionals. Schedule a time with your doctor when you can discuss your fears and frustrations and find answers to your questions about the condition. You might also consider joining a support group. Organizations such as the Crohn's & Colitis Foundation of America (CCFA) have chapters across the country. Medical professionals also can help you locate the local chapter or you can contact the organization directly. (See also "Additional resources" on pages 241-244.)

Some people find it helpful to consult a psychologist or psychiatrist regarding their anxieties. Try to locate a professional who's familiar with inflammatory bowel disease and who understands some of the emotional difficulties it produces.

Surgery

For most people with IBD, treatment with medication or changes in lifestyle provide a significant improvement of signs and symptoms. But some people eventually decide on surgery to treat their condition.

With Crohn's disease, removal of the damaged portion of the small intestine or colon can provide years of relief. During the procedure, healthy sections of intestine are reconnected after the damaged portion is removed. The surgeon may also close fistulas and remove scar tissue that's blocking the intestinal passage.

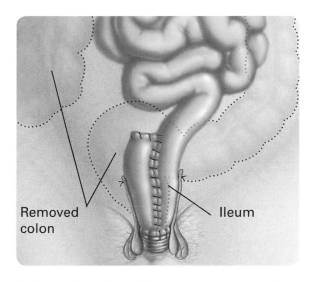

Removed colon

Ileum

In ileoanal anastomosis, a surgeon removes the colon and innermost lining of the rectum, creates a J-shaped pouch out of the last section of the small intestine (ileum), then reattaches the pouch near the anal sphincter. Leaving the anal sphincter and rectal muscles intact allows near-normal passage of stool.

Laparoscopic surgery requires much smaller incisions than traditional surgery does, and shorter recovery times. But often, surgery doesn't cure the disease. It simply returns at other locations in your digestive tract.

Ulcerative colitis is different — surgery can cure the disease. Unfortunately, the procedure often requires complete removal of the colon and rectum. About 20 to 25 percent undergo surgery because of continual bleeding, severe illness or risk of cancer.

Two options

Surgery to remove the colon and rectum is call proctocolectomy (prok-toh-koh-LEK-tuh-me). Using the traditional approach to this surgery, an opening (stoma) about the size of a quarter is made in the lower right corner of the abdomen, near the belt-line. After removal of the colon and rectum, the last portion of the small intestine (ileum) is attached to the stoma.

A small bag (ileostomy bag) is worn over the stoma to collect waste. Periodic emptying of the bag is needed. This surgery is used mainly for older people who don't have good control of the anal sphincter muscle.

A procedure used for many people with ulcerative colitis eliminates the need to wear an ileostomy bag. Called ileoanal anastomosis, this two-stage surgery takes advantage of the fact that inflammation associated with ulcerative colitis generally doesn't involve deep tissues of the intestines. (See the illustration on page 157.)

The surgeon removes your colon and the innermost lining of your rectum. A small J-shaped pouch is constructed from the end of your small intestine (ileum) and is attached directly to the anus and supported by remaining layers of rectal tissue. Waste will be stored in the pouch and expelled normally, though bowel movements are more frequent and watery. On average, you may have four to six loose bowel movements a day.

During the first stage of surgery, a temporary ileostomy — when the small intestine is attached to an opening in the abdominal wall — is created. This diverts feces away from the ileal pouch until the new area of intestine has had time to heal. Feces collects in an external bag, similar to what happens in a proctocolectomy. The ileostomy is removed during a second operation that usually takes place about three months after the first.

Ileoanal anastomosis surgery is usually done through a long incision across the midline of the abdomen. However, some specially trained surgeons perform this procedure laparoscopically, which helps to shorten hospital stays and recovery time. Some people develop inflammation in their pouch (pouchitis) after this operation. Usually, this can be treated with antibiotics or other medications.

Chapter 9

Celiac disease

You may have noticed problems that started with a viral infection or during pregnancy or while you were experiencing a period of high stress. You began to struggle with intermittent bouts of diarrhea and bloating and weight loss. Now, weeks or months later, the signs and symptoms continue, even after the infection has cleared up, the pregnancy ended or your stressful situation resolved itself. You're living, eating and exercising much as you always did. What's happened?

The signs and symptoms may be occurring because the initial condition — be it from infection, pregnancy, stress or some form of trauma — has triggered onset of a second condition, a lifelong intestinal disorder known as celiac (SEE-lee-ak) disease.

Key signs and symptoms

- Diarrhea
- Abdominal gas
- Bloating
- Fatigue
- Weight loss
- Stunted growth (in children)
- Osteoporosis
- Anemia

Celiac disease damages the interior of the small intestine and interferes with its ability to absorb certain nutrients from food. People with celiac disease can't tolerate gluten, a protein found in many products made of wheat, barley, rye and some oats.

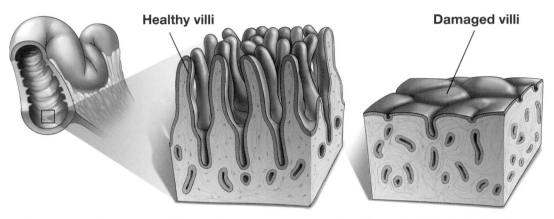

Healthy villi   Damaged villi

The inner surface of a healthy small intestine is lined with millions of villi (left). Celiac disease damages the villi, causing them to shrink and disappear (right). This affects your body's ability to absorb nutrients from the food you eat, leading to malnutrition and other illnesses.

In fact, gluten can be found in common grain products that are prepared and eaten every day, including bread, pasta, pizza crust, cookies, cakes and pastries. (Products made with corn or rice flour do not contain gluten and are safe to eat if you have celiac disease.)

If you have celiac disease and you eat something that contains gluten, an immune reaction inflames and swells the inner lining of your small intestine. The inflammation causes tiny hair-like projections (villi) in the small intestine to shrink and even disappear.

Normally, your small intestine is lined with millions of villi (VIL-i), resembling the deep pile of a plush carpet on a microscopic scale. The villi work to absorb nutrients from the food you eat.

When celiac disease damages villi, the inner surface of your small intestine becomes less like a plush carpet and more like a tile floor. Your body is unable to absorb many essential nutrients necessary for good health. Instead, fat, protein, vitamins and minerals are eliminated from your body via your stool.

Over time, poor absorption (malabsorption) affects your brain, nerves, bones, liver and other organs. The result is often malnutrition and may lead to other illnesses. No treatment can cure celiac disease, but you can effectively manage the disease through diet.

Celiac disease, also known as celiac sprue, nontropical sprue and gluten sensitive enteropathy, is one of many different malabsorption disorders.

The cause of celiac disease is unknown but it's often inherited. If someone in your immediate family has it, there's a higher chance that you may as well.

Celiac disease affects about 1 in 133 people in the United States. It can occur at any age, and it tends to be more common in people of European descent and people with other autoimmune disorders, such as lupus erythematosus, type 1 diabetes, rheumatoid arthritis or autoimmune thyroid disease.

Some people first notice the signs and symptoms as children, others as adults. Many times, for reasons that aren't clear, the disease emerges after some form of trauma, such as an infection, physical injury, the stress of pregnancy, severe stress or surgery. How or why these conditions trigger the onset of celiac disease is unclear.

Signs and symptoms

Celiac disease may date back thousands of years, but it has been only in the last 50 years that researchers have gained a better understanding of the condition and how to treat it.

There is no typical form of the disease. Some people exhibit little or no signs and symptoms and may live with celiac disease for years before it's diagnosed. For other people, the signs and symptoms vary and may include fatigue, abdominal pain, intermittent diarrhea, bloating, nausea, weight loss and excessive passing of gas.

Fatigue can result from a sharp reduction of red blood cells in your bloodstream (anemia). Other indications of malabsorption are weight loss and lighter colored, foul-smelling stools.

Celiac disease may also present itself in less obvious ways, including changes in behavior such as irritability or depression, joint pain, muscle cramps, skin rash, mouth sores, dental and bone disorders, infertility, tingling in the legs, and delayed growth in children.

When you have celiac disease, you usually have higher than normal levels of antibodies to gluten circulating in your bloodstream. Tests that measure anti-gliadin antibodies (AGAs), anti-endomysial antibodies (EMAs) and tissue transglutaminase antibodies (tTGs) can detect celiac disease at an early stage. The test for tTG antibodies has proved particularly effective, identifying celiac disease in most cases.

If your signs and symptoms, and blood test results, suggest celiac disease, your doctor may remove a small tissue sample (biopsy) from your small intestine and examine it under a microscope for damaged villi. Generally, the sample is obtained by threading a thin, flexible tube (endoscope) through your upper gastrointestinal tract and into the small intestine (see pages 84-86).

One way that may help confirm celiac disease after diagnostic testing is if your signs and symptoms improve by eliminating gluten from your diet.

However, don't go on a gluten-free diet without first consulting your doctor. Doing so may create false negatives, making the results of blood tests and biopsies appear normal.

Some people who don't have celiac disease develop similar signs and symptoms, such as gas, bloating, abdominal discomfort and loose stools. This happens because they're intolerant of wheat — a situation similar to people who develop lactose intolerance (see pages 58-59). The wheat is not completely digested in the small intestine

Similar but different diseases

Several conditions may cause malabsorption with signs and symptoms that resemble celiac disease. They include tropical sprue, Whipple's disease, giardiasis infection, bacterial overgrowth and immunoglobulin deficiency. Your doctor often can identify special features that distinguish these conditions from celiac disease. In addition, they don't respond to a gluten-free diet.

Dermatitis herpetiformis is an itchy, blistering skin disease that also stems from gluten intolerance. The rash usually occurs on the elbows, knees and buttocks. Dermatitis herpetiformis can cause significant intestinal damage that's identical to celiac disease. However, it may not produce noticeable digestive signs and symptoms. The disease is treated with a gluten-free diet, in addition to medication to control the rash.

and passed into the colon, where bacteria ferment it, producing gas and loose stool. This condition is distinct from celiac disease, which involves a reaction to gluten, an element in wheat as well as certain other types of grain.

New way of eating

Celiac disease is a chronic condition, and there are no medications or medical procedures such as surgery that can cure it. The focus of treatment is on relieving signs and symptoms while allowing you to maintain a varied, balanced and nutritious diet.

Managing the disease and preventing its complications will likely require you to change or adapt the types of food you eat. It's critical that you avoid gluten. That means avoiding all foods or food ingredients made from the grains wheat, barley and rye.

Whether or not people with celiac disease can safely eat oats is controversial. Several studies suggest that eating moderate amounts of oats had no harmful effects on the inner lining of the small intestine. However, some experts continue to be concerned that oats can be harmful.

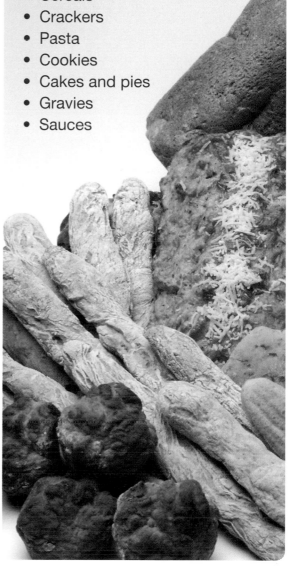

Foods that contain gluten

Most foods made from grains contain gluten. Avoid these foods unless they're made with corn or rice or labeled as gluten-free.

- Breads
- Cereals
- Crackers
- Pasta
- Cookies
- Cakes and pies
- Gravies
- Sauces

Food ingredients that contain gluten

Avoid all food products that list any of the following as ingredients.

- Wheat (wheat flour, white flour, wheat bran, wheat germ, farina, wheat starch, graham flour, semolina, durum)
- Barley
- Rye
- Oats (oat flour, oat bran, oatmeal)
- Bulgur
- Kasha
- Khorasan wheat
- Matzo meal
- Spelt
- Triticale

New grain-containing products appear on the market periodically. Avoid them until you can verify their safety from a reliable source, such as a dietitian.

When you first make dietary changes, you may also need to take vitamin and mineral supplements recommended by your doctor or a dietitian to help correct nutritional deficiencies. As your symptoms subside and your ability to absorb nutrients improves, the need for supplements may diminish. If you have osteoporosis due to celiac disease, you may need to continue taking calcium and vitamin D supplements long term.

Within just a few days of removing gluten from your diet, the inflammation in your small intestine will likely begin to subside. It can take from several months to two to three years for your intestine to heal completely.

Getting used to your new diet can be difficult. It may take several months to sort out which foods you can or can't eat. You may crave certain foods that you're no longer allowed to eat. But don't get discouraged and give up. With time, most people learn to adjust to a gluten-free diet, and it becomes a normal part of their daily life.

If you accidentally eat a food product that contains gluten, you may or may not experience abdominal pain and diarrhea. Trace amounts of gluten in your diet still can be damaging to the villi in your intestinal tract. Over time, these small amounts may increase your risk of many serious complications, including anemia, osteoporosis, seizures, lymphoma or cancer of the small intestine, and in children, stunted growth and development.

Risks of gluten in your diet

Many processed foods include an ingredient or ingredients that contain gluten, so it's important to always check food labels — particularly with a new product that you may be unfamiliar with. However, you can't always tell by reading a food label whether the product is gluten-free.

For example, hydrolyzed vegetable protein (HVP) may appear in the list of ingredients, but the label usually doesn't indicate whether the HVP is made from soy, corn or wheat. Therefore, it's not safe for you to eat the food. HVP that comes from wheat would include gluten, whereas you would be safe with HVP from soy or corn.

In general, avoid all processed foods unless you can verify from the manufacturer that none of the ingredients contains gluten. (See "Reading food labels" on page 167.)

Eating a gluten-free diet

When you hear that the treatment for celiac disease is a gluten-free diet, you may feel at first that your food choices have been severely restricted. Take heart that there is a wide variety of nutritious, tasty foods that don't contain gluten. With time and patience, mixed with a little creativity and a willingness to explore new options, you can find many common foods to enjoy.

Base your diet on a foundation of fresh vegetables and fruits, which are naturally gluten-free. It's more challenging

Sources of support

Many professionals can help you adjust to a gluten-free diet. Your doctor and a registered dietitian are first on the list. A support group for people with celiac disease may even exist in your community.

Several national organizations also provide support services, including diet information. See "Additional resources" beginning on page 241.

Surprising sources of gluten

You may ingest gluten in ways that you would never expect. Common examples are through cross-contamination, when gluten-free foods come in contact with foods containing gluten. This may happen if you share a knife for spreading butter that has bread crumbs on it, use the same toaster as others, or eat deep-fried foods that are cooked in the same oil used for breaded foods. Nonedible products also may contain gluten, including:

- Certain medications (which use gluten as a binding agent)
- Lipstick
- Postage stamps
- Communion wafers

Your best bet is to contact the manufacturers of these products to find out if they contain gluten. Allow a pharmacist to inspect containers for each medication you take. In the case of stamps, use the self-adhesive kind.

whenever you buy packaged foods at the grocery store, order at a restaurant, or consider a snack at social events and parties. A balanced diet that's gluten-free can include foods such as:

- Plain meats (not breaded or marinated)
- Fruits
- Vegetables
- Pasta from corn, rice and other gluten-free grains
- Quinoa
- Rice, including cereal and crackers made from rice

- Potatoes and potato flour
- Most dairy products
- Tapioca
- Amaranth
- Buckwheat

There are many gluten-free flours to choose from if you make breads, cakes and other foods. Be aware that gluten-free grains can be contaminated with gluten-containing grains. This can happen, inadvertently, during harvesting, transporting or processing. Check that the label indicates the flour is gluten-free, or that the manufacturer ensures that it is.

Celiac disease and lactose intolerance

Because of the damage to your small intestine from gluten, foods that don't contain gluten also may cause abdominal pain and diarrhea. For example, some people with celiac disease aren't able to tolerate the lactose found in dairy products — a condition known as lactose intolerance. In addition to avoiding gluten, these people also must limit food and drink containing lactose.

After your small intestine has healed, you may be able to tolerate dairy products once again. However, lactose intolerance may continue despite your successful management of celiac disease. If that's the case, you'll need to limit or avoid most dairy products for the rest of your life.

A dietitian can help you plan a diet that's low in lactose as well as gluten-free. If you can no longer eat dairy products, it's important that you find other sources of calcium.

If you don't enjoy the kitchen, you can purchase ready-made products that are gluten-free. A registered dietitian can help you locate these products. Local or national celiac disease support groups also can be helpful. Some have published lists of commercially produced or packaged items that don't contain gluten, to help you with shopping.

Contact the Tri-County Celiac Support Group or Celiac Sprue Association for copies of these shopping guides. Make sure they have been updated within the past two years.

Read food labels

Food labels are important tools for making safe food choices when you have celiac disease. Always read the food label before purchasing any product. Some foods that seem acceptable, such as rice or corn cereals, may actually contain small amounts of gluten.

A manufacturer may change a product's ingredients at any time without announcing it. A food that was once gluten-free may no longer be. Unless you read the label, you won't know.

If you can't tell by the label if a food includes gluten, don't eat it until you get that information from a gluten-free shopper's guide or the product's manufacturer. It's a good idea to check with manufacturers periodically to be sure the information you have is current.

Eating out

Preparing your own meals is the best way to ensure your diet is gluten-free. But that doesn't mean that you can't eat out on occasion. These guidelines can help you have a safe dining experience:

- Select a restaurant that specializes in the kinds of foods you can eat. You may call the restaurant in advance to discuss its menu options.
- Visit the same restaurants so that you become familiar with their menus and so the personnel get to know your needs.

- Ask members of your support group for suggestions on restaurants that serve gluten-free food.
- Follow the same practices you do at home. Select simply prepared or fresh foods and avoid all breaded or batter-coated foods.

When diet isn't enough

Most people with celiac disease who follow a gluten-free diet can return to normal health within a few weeks. A small percentage who experience severe damage in their small intestines don't improve with a gluten-free diet.

When diet isn't effective, treatment often includes medications to control intestinal inflammation and other conditions resulting from malabsorption. Because celiac disease is a lifelong condition, it's important to see your doctor regularly to monitor your health.

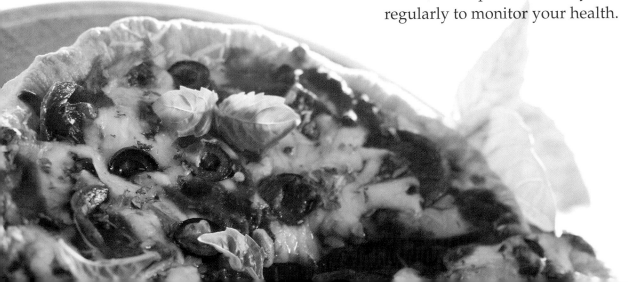

Chapter 10

Diverticular disease

Many people develop small, bulging pouches in the organs of their digestive tract, particularly as they age. These pouches vary in size. They form when the inner layer of tissue in the organ walls pushes through weak spots in the outer layer, resembling a series of small balloons bulging outward.

Each pouch is called a diverticulum (di-vur-TIK-u-lum), from Latin words meaning "a small diversion from the normal path." The name for more than one diverticulum is *diverticula*.

Diverticula can form anywhere in your digestive tract, including the throat, esophagus, stomach and small intestine. But the most common location is your large intestine (colon), particularly on the left side in sections known as the descending colon and sigmoid colon.

The general term for this condition is diverticular disease. Diverticula by themselves generally don't cause problems, but sometimes the pouches become inflamed or infected. You'll need to contact your doctor when they start causing severe abdominal pain.

Key signs and symptoms

- Pain in the lower left abdomen
- Abdominal tenderness
- Fever
- Nausea
- Constipation or diarrhea

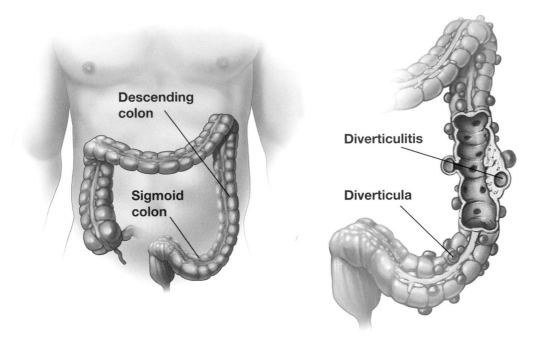

The most common locations for small pouches (diverticula) to form is in the descending and sigmoid sections of the colon. When a pouch becomes inflamed or infected, the condition is called diverticulitis. In the endoscopic image of the colon below, diverticula are evident in the intestinal walls.

Diverticulosis

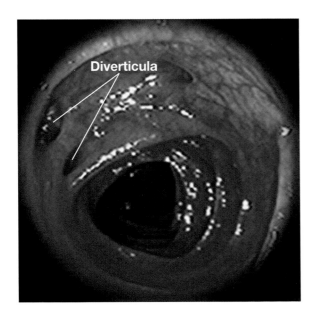

Whenever diverticula form in your digestive tract, the condition is called diverticulosis. The pouches — which are often about the size of a marble — ordinarily don't cause any problems, and many people with the condition don't even know they have it.

Diverticulosis is relatively common and becomes more prevalent as you get older. Nearly half the Americans older than age 60 have diverticula somewhere along their digestive tracts, most often in their colons.

When a pouch bleeds

A few people with diverticulosis will experience painless rectal bleeding. The blood may be dark and mixed with stool, but more often it is bright red and plainly visible in the toilet bowl. Usually the result of a weakened blood vessel that has burst, the bleeding can be sudden and severe, requiring immediate medical attention.

Bleeding from a ruptured blood vessel in a diverticulum is typically short-lived and often stops by itself, without treatment. If the bleeding is severe or persistent, you may need tests to identify the location of the bleeding. Occasionally, surgery is necessary to remove a segment of the colon where the bleeding pouch is located, as the only way to stop the bleeding.

A minority of people with diverticulosis experience mild abdominal cramps, bloating, gas, diarrhea or constipation. However, these signs and symptoms are more likely related to other conditions, such as irritable bowel syndrome, and not to diverticulosis. Bleeding isn't typically a sign of diverticulosis, but it can occur in some people (see "When a pouch bleeds" sidebar above).

Diverticulitis

When inflammation or infection develops in a diverticulum, the condition becomes known as diverticulitis. Some people experience only minor inflammation, while others have a massive, painful infection. A cause of diverticulitis may be a small portion of stool becoming trapped in one of the pouches. The stool blocks blood supply to the pouch and makes it susceptible to the invasion of bacteria. A small tear (perforation) also can develop in a diverticulum, leading to infection and, sometimes, a collection of pus.

Generally, inflammation or infection is limited to the area directly around the diverticulum. In rare cases, the pouch ruptures through a large perforation, spilling intestinal waste into your abdominal cavity. This can lead to peritonitis (per-ih-toe-NI-tis), an inflammation of the thin membrane that lines the abdominal cavity. This condition is usually very painful and often accompanied by fever and chills. Peritonitis is a medical emergency that demands immediate attention to fight the infection and treat the underlying condition.

Diverticulitis typically causes pain, fever, chills and nausea. The pain often is abrupt and severe, but some people experience mild pain that gradually worsens over several days.

Symptoms of diverticulitis are similar in many ways to those of appendicitis, except that the pain is usually in the lower left side of your abdomen, instead of the lower right side. Less common signs and symptoms include vomiting, bloating, rectal bleeding, frequent urination, and difficulty or pain while urinating.

Pressure problems

The reasons why some people develop diverticula in their digestive tract while others don't isn't well understood. The trigger appears to be strong pressure that's exerted within the digestive tract. This pressure forces inner layers of tissue to bulge outward through weak spots in the outer layers. Three factors seem to play roles in this process:

Weak spots in colon wall

The colon is ringed by layers of muscle that regularly relax and contract (peristalsis). This action helps propel food waste through the digestive tract to the rectum. Blood vessels penetrate natural defects in the outer layers of the colon walls to deliver essential nutrients to the inner layers. These locations are structurally weaker than the rest of the colon wall.

When, for example, you strain to pass stool, you increase the pressure within your colon. This pressure can cause the inner tissue to bulge out through these weak spots, forming diverticula.

Aging

Research suggests that as you age, the outer wall of muscle in your colon begins to thicken, causing the inner passage of the colon to narrow. This narrowing increases the level of pressure in your colon, which also raises the risk of pouch formation.

Thickening of the outer wall also makes the colon less flexible and able to move food waste quickly. Waste stays in the colon longer, where it exerts pressure on the inner layers of tissue.

Too little fiber

Technological improvements in industrial societies also seem to have played a role with diverticular disease. The disease was first observed in the United States in the early 1900s — around the time that steel rolling mills were introduced into the flour-milling process. The new process greatly reduced the fiber content of flour and other grain-derived foods that are mainstays in the American diet.

Today, diverticular disease is more common in industrialized nations, such as the United States and in Western Europe, where the average diet is high in refined carbohydrates and low in fiber. In countries where people eat a high-fiber diet, often in places that are not as industrialized, the disease is rare.

Too little fiber in your diet contributes to small, hard stools or soft, mushy stools that are difficult to pass through your intestinal tract. This increases the pressure in your colon, and the highest pressures occur in the sigmoid colon, where most diverticula are found.

Don't worry about seeds

You may have heard that eating foods containing seeds, such as raspberries, strawberries or kiwis, is dangerous because the tiny seeds can become lodged in a diverticulum and cause inflammation or infection.

Recent research has found these foods weren't associated with an increased risk of diverticulitis. In addition, it's questionable to forgo healthy fruits and vegetables that contain seeds for fear of infection. The nutrients and fiber these foods provide outweigh any increased risk of diverticulitis.

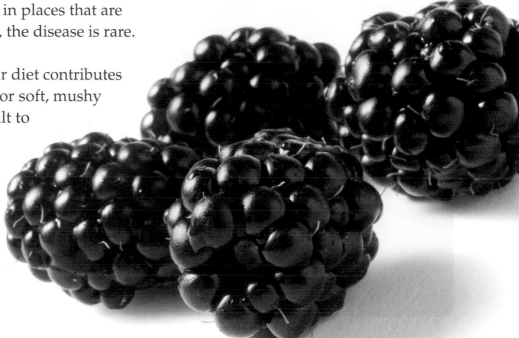

Diagnosis

Because the presence of diverticula alone generally doesn't cause signs and symptoms, most people learn they have diverticulosis during routine screening exams for colorectal cancer or during testing to determine the cause of various intestinal problems. Imaging tests such as colonoscopy, sigmoidoscopy, computerized tomography (CT) or colon X-ray may reveal one or more of the pouches. For more on these imaging procedures, see Chapter 4.

Diverticulitis, on the other hand, is typically diagnosed during an acute episode when signs and symptoms such as abdominal pain, fever and nausea compel you to see a doctor. The doctor will check your abdomen for areas of tenderness. You may receive a blood test for your white blood cell count. An elevated number of white blood cells and tenderness in the lower left abdomen may signal diverticulitis.

Imaging tests such as a CT scan may help detect the inflammation or infection and confirm the diagnosis. During acute episodes of diverticulitis, tests such as colonoscopy, sigmoidoscopy, barium enema and CT colonography should not be performed.

Treatment begins with self-care

The key to managing diverticular disease is reducing the pressure inside your colon. Often, this can be accomplished with routine steps you take at home. Although signs and symptoms of diverticulosis are rare, it's still important to establish daily habits that keep your digestive tract healthy and functioning smoothly. These measures may prevent or reduce the formation of new diverticula.

Treating diverticulitis will depend on how severe your signs and symptoms are and on whether this is your first attack or not. If signs and symptoms are mild, you may be able to treat the condition with changes to your diet and possibly a course of antibiotics to fight the infection.

If you're having recurrent attacks of diverticulitis or you're at risk of complications, you may need more advanced treatment requiring medication or surgery. Complications include bowel obstruction and peritonitis.

The following are self-care steps for managing diverticular disease:

Eat more fiber

High-fiber foods, such as fresh fruits and vegetables and whole-grain products, soften stool and help it pass more quickly through the colon. This reduces pressure inside your digestive tract and helps prevent episodes of diverticulitis.

Depending on your age and sex, aim for 21 to 38 grams of fiber each day. (See "Where to find fiber" on pages 33-34 for a list of high-fiber foods.) Try to substitute fruits, vegetables and grain products for foods high in fat.

People with mild signs and symptoms of diverticular disease often find that after a week or two of eating more fiber their condition begins to improve. However, avoid a sudden, large increase in dietary fiber. This can lead to gas, cramping, bloating and diarrhea. Gradually increasing fiber over several weeks usually works best.

If you find it difficult to consume the recommended amount of fiber each day, talk to your doctor about regular use of a natural fiber supplement. These include over-the-counter products such as psyllium (Metamucil) and methylcellulose (Citrucel). These products generally help relieve constipation within weeks, and can also help prevent constipation.

Drink plenty of fluids

Fiber acts as a sponge in your colon, absorbing water into stool. As you increase the amount of fiber you eat, make sure you also drink plenty of liquid to replace the lost fluid and prevent constipation. Each day, drink at least eight 8-ounce glasses of water or other beverages that don't contain caffeine or alcohol. For more on fluids, see page 35.

Respond to bowel urges

Anytime you need to pass stool, don't delay a trip to the bathroom. Delaying a bowel movement leads to harder stools, requiring more force and increasing pressure within your colon.

Exercise regularly

Exercise promotes normal bowel function and reduces pressure inside your colon. Try to exercise for 30 to 60 minutes on most days of the week. For more information on the value of exercise, see pages 43-46.

If self-care is not enough

Acute episodes of diverticulitis signal the development of inflammation or infection in one of the diverticula. When that happens, treatment will generally require more than self-care. Depending on how severe your symptoms are, you may be hospitalized or you may be treated at home. About half the people with diverticulitis, including those with vomiting, fever, high white blood cell count, or possible bowel obstruction, or people who are at risk of peritonitis, will require hospitalization.

You're also more likely to be hospitalized if you're older, are taking steroids, have another disease or have a weakened immune system.

Nonsurgical treatments for diverticulitis include:

Rest and restricted diet

A few days of rest allows the infection time to heal. A liquid diet or low-fiber diet reduces the number of contractions in your colon, which aids healing. In case of severe nausea and vomiting, you may have to avoid all food and take fluids intravenously.

Once your symptoms improve — often in two to four days — you can begin eating more foods, gradually building up to a high-fiber diet.

Antibiotics

Antibiotics kill bacteria causing the infection. It's important to continue taking the full course of an antibiotic, even if you feel better after a few days. Follow the prescription exactly as your doctor or pharmacist has advised.

Painkillers

If your symptoms are accompanied by moderate to severe pain, your doctor may recommend an over-the-counter or prescription analgesic for a few days until the pain improves. These nonsurgical practices — rest, diet, antibiotics and possibly a painkiller — often are effective treatment for a first attack of diverticulitis. Unfortunately, recurrent episodes are less likely to respond to simple measures and may require more advanced care.

The likelihood of you having more than one episode of diverticulitis varies. For most people, the risk of recurrence after one attack is about 25 percent. You can help prevent a second attack by eating more fiber, drinking plenty of liquids and getting plenty of exercise. After a second attack, the risk of recurrence is over 50 percent.

Surgery for diverticulitis

If one of the following complications from diverticulitis occurs, surgery may be needed to treat your condition:

- Peritonitis, which occurs if a ruptured pouch spills its contents into your abdominal cavity
- Blockage in your colon or small intestine caused by scar tissue
- Formation of an abscess when pus collects in a pouch
- Formation of a fistula, which is an abnormal passageway between two organs, such as the colon and bladder, resulting from disease in one of the organs

Peritonitis requires emergency surgery. Often a temporary colostomy is required that includes a bag worn outside the body to collect stool. (For more on this procedure, see page 178.)

Other problems, such as narrowing of the colon or formation of a fistula, may require surgery after the inflammation has subsided, usually about six to eight weeks after the attack.

An abscess can be drained, often without surgery, by a radiologist using an X-ray-guided needle to collect the pus. This procedure can take place at the time of the attack. However, surgery may still be needed six to eight weeks later to prevent a recurrence.

To prevent future infections, doctors often recommend that people with recurring diverticulitis have surgery to remove the diseased portion of the colon. There are two forms of surgery:

Primary bowel resection
This procedure is standard for people with diverticulitis who don't need emergency surgery. The surgeon removes the diseased part of your colon and then reconnects the remaining, healthy segments (anastomosis). This keeps your colon passage open and allows normal bowel movements.

The extent of the inflammation in your colon and other complicating factors, such as obesity, help determine whether you're a candidate for traditional surgery or laparoscopic surgery.

With traditional surgery, the surgeon makes one long incision in your abdomen. With laparoscopic surgery, three or four small incisions are made. Laparoscopic surgery requires less recovery time, but generally it isn't possible for people who are obese or who have extensive inflammation or infection.

Bowel resection with colostomy

This surgical procedure may be necessary if you have so much inflammation that it's not possible to rejoin your colon and rectum. A colostomy will allow you to continue eliminating stool from your body.

During the procedure, called Hartmann's procedure, a surgeon removes the diseased section of colon, closes off the upper part of the rectum and makes an opening in your abdominal wall. The colon is connected to this opening to create the colostomy. Stool passes through the opening and into a bag attached to the abdominal wall.

A colostomy may be temporary or permanent. Several months later — after the inflammation has healed — your doctor may consider a second operation to reconnect the colon and rectum. It's important that you discuss with your doctor the benefits and risks of such an operation.

Is there cancer risk?

There's no evidence that diverticulosis or diverticulitis increases your risk of colon or rectal cancer, or the formation of precancerous growths (polyps) in the lining of the colon or rectum. However, diverticular disease can make cancer more difficult to diagnose.

After an episode of diverticulitis, your doctor may suggest a colonoscopy or another screening test to make sure that you don't have cancer or some other inflammatory disease of the colon or rectum. The screening test can be done several weeks after the episode, allowing time for healing.

Chapter 11

Gallstones

It's bedtime, but you can't sleep. There's persistent pain in your upper abdomen and nothing relieves it — not antacids and not pain relievers. Changing your position doesn't help. You stand up, bend over, lie down, but the pain stays. Then, you start feeling nauseated. When pain spreads to the lower chest and back, you visit the emergency room, worried about a heart attack.

At the hospital, you learn that the problem is not your heart but your gallbladder. Pain develops when hard, pebble-sized deposits, or "stones," become lodged in the neck of the gallbladder, the narrow portion of the organ that connects to the cystic duct. This obstruction blocks the flow of bile, which builds pressure in the gallbladder and causes pain and often nausea.

Key signs and symptoms

- Upper abdominal pain
- Pain in back, chest or right shoulder blade
- Nausea and vomiting

Gallstones are common. Ten to 15 percent of Americans have them. For most people, they cause no symptoms and require no treatment. But many people with gallstones will experience painful attacks. Gallbladder attacks account for one of the most common operations in the United States — gallbladder removal (cholecystectomy). Thousands of Americans have their gallbladders removed each year.

How gallstones form

Your gallbladder is a pear-shaped sac about 3 to 6 inches long and 1 to 2 inches across at its widest point. It's tucked under the liver, on the right side of your upper abdomen. The gallbladder is part of the biliary system that includes the liver and an intricate network of ducts for transporting bile.

Bile is a digestive fluid produced in your liver. The gallbladder serves as a reservoir for bile until it's ready for use in the small intestine. The composition of bile includes bilirubin (bil-ih-ROO-bin), a greenish-yellow waste product from the liver that gives the fluid its

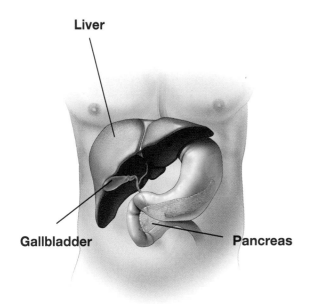

Liver

Gallbladder   **Pancreas**

color. That's why, if bile backs up into your blood, it can cause your skin and eyes to turn yellow (jaundice).

Bile also contains cholesterol, bile salts and the chemical lecithin (LES-ih-thin). Together, the bile salts and lecithin keep cholesterol dissolved in solution, allowing it to be excreted out of your body.

But the primary function of bile is helping break down fat molecules in the food you eat. Fat is a source of valuable nutrients and, without the action of bile, these nutrients would be flushed out of your system as waste.

When you eat a meal containing fat or protein — which likely means most of your meals — your gallbladder takes action. The organ contracts and empties the bile it holds in reserve through small tubes called bile ducts, which lead to your upper small intestine (duodenum). Once in the duodenum, bile helps your small intestine digest and absorb fat and the fat-soluble vitamins, A, D, E and K.

When bile becomes chemically imbalanced, it forms into hardened particles, which can grow into stones as small as a grain of sand or bigger than a golf ball. Some people have just one stone, while others have multiple stones that may number in the hundreds or even thousands, sometimes referred to as gravel, sand or sludge.

Multiple factors may contribute to the formation of gallstones, many of which aren't well understood, including:

Too much cholesterol

Normally, your bile contains enough chemicals to dissolve the cholesterol excreted by your liver. But if your bile contains more cholesterol than can be dissolved, the extra cholesterol can form eventually into stones. Obesity, genetics — for example, American Indian heritage — and rapid weight loss may contribute to this process.

Gallbladder doesn't empty correctly

Your gallbladder may fail to contract and empty as it should. This may occur during pregnancy or from prolonged fasting. The longer bile stays in your gallbladder, the more concentrated it becomes. Bile that's too concentrated can become sludgy and form stones.

Too much bilirubin

Certain conditions, such as liver cirrhosis, may cause too much of the chemical bilirubin to be in bile. Too much bilirubin may contribute to the formation of gallstones.

Types of stones

Not all gallstones have the same composition. You may have one of the following varieties:

Cholesterol stones

The most common type of gallstone is composed primarily of cholesterol produced in your liver that bile is unable to keep dissolved. They often contain other components and usually appear yellow in color.

Pigment stones

This type of stone forms when bile contains too much bilirubin. Pigment stones are generally small and dark brown or black in color. Some are associated with excess production of

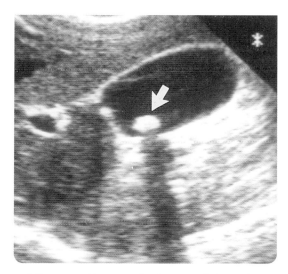

Ultrasound image of a large gallstone (arrow) inside the gallbladder

bilirubin due to excessive red blood cell destruction, and others from severe scarring of the liver (cirrhosis).

Primary bile duct stones

Stones that escape from the gallbladder and lodge in the bile ducts are known as secondary or retained duct stones.

Primary bile duct stones actually form in the bile ducts. The stones are usually

soft and brown, made of decomposed bile, and occur when a bile duct is narrowed because of infection or strictures due to trauma, surgery or disease.

Gallstone attack

Gallstones usually settle at the bottom of your gallbladder, and most of the time they don't cause problems. Some people associate gallstones with certain signs and symptoms, such as heartburn, indigestion or bloating. However, there's no evidence that gallbladder disease causes these problems.

It's when the stones migrate up to the neck (outlet) of the gallbladder that problems may occur. When your gallbladder expels bile into the biliary system, some of the stones may be carried along with the fluid.

The smallest stones usually pass through the bile ducts, enter the small intestine and leave your body without incident. But larger gallstones can get stuck at the entrance to the cystic duct, within a bile duct or at the entrance to the small intestine.

When a gallstone blocks the flow of bile from the gallbladder, it can cause nausea and steady pain that may be

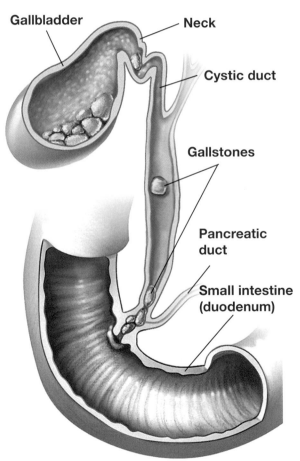

Gallbladder
Neck
Cystic duct
Gallstones
Pancreatic duct
Small intestine (duodenum)

A gallstone attack may occur wherever stones become lodged in a bile duct.

moderate to severe (biliary pain or biliary colic). This is what's known as a gallbladder attack. The attack may last from 15 minutes to several hours.

Usually, a stone lodged at the entrance to the cystic duct will drop back down to the bottom of your gallbladder. That reopens the passage and generally signals the end of the attack. If the stone doesn't work its way free, inflammation and infection may occur within the gallbladder (cholecystitis).

Other signs and symptoms of a gallbladder attack may include fever, chills, nausea and vomiting.

Other complications of gallstones may occur. They happen if:

- The cystic duct remains blocked, and infection causes the gallbladder to rupture, although rupture is rare
- A stone lodged in a duct blocks bile flow from the liver, which may cause jaundice, as well as fever, chills and blood infection such as sepsis, bacteremia or cholangitis
- Gallstones that collect at the entrance to the small intestine — usually for a short amount of time — block the pancreatic duct, causing inflammation of the pancreas (pancreatitis)

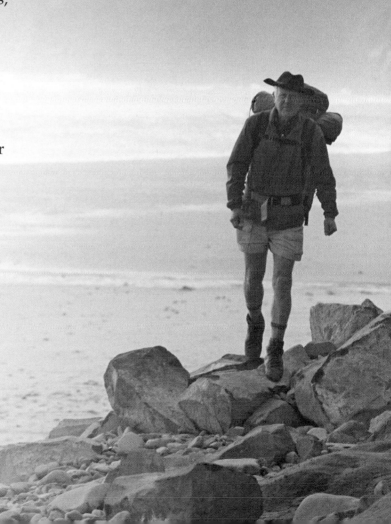

Are you at risk?

The reasons why gallstones develop in some people and not in others remain unclear. The following factors may put you at increased risk:

Being female
Gallstones are twice as common in women as in men. That may be because of the hormone estrogen, an essential element in the female reproductive system, which exists in much higher amounts in women than in men.

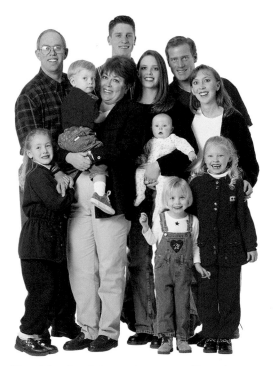

The risk of gallstones increases if you're female — women are twice as likely as men to have them. But gallstones also tend to run in families, regardless of age or sex.

Estrogen causes the liver to excrete more cholesterol into your bile, increasing the likelihood of stone formation.

Pregnancy, birth control pills and hormone replacement therapy also increase the level of cholesterol in bile, and decrease your gallbladder's ability to completely empty bile. However, you shouldn't stop taking birth control pills or hormone replacement therapy simply out of concern. Consult your doctor first. The benefits may outweigh any increased risk of gallstones.

Family history
Gallstones often run in families, pointing to a possible genetic link. Recent studies have identified two genes associated with an increased risk of gallstones, regardless of the age, sex or weight of the carrier.

Ethnic group
Native Americans have the highest incidence of gallstones in the United States, followed by people of Hispanic origin — many of whom have some Native American heritage. Among Pima Indians of Arizona, more than 70 percent of females have gallstones by age 30, and most males eventually have them. People of Asian or African descent are among the least likely to have gallstones.

Can you prevent gallstones?

Some home remedies recommend drinking olive oil, apple juice or lemon juice to stimulate your gallbladder to empty out small stones. However, these practices have demonstrated no beneficial effect.

The fact is there is no diet shown to prevent gallstones. But there are two steps you can take that may lower your risk. One is to maintain a healthy weight. The other is to avoid extreme diets that involve a low intake of calories and rapid weight loss.

Although not scientifically proved, there's some indication that exercise may help prevent gallstones. Researchers speculate that physical activity may help stabilize the delicate chemical balance of bile, helping to keep cholesterol dissolved in solution and inhibiting the formation of stones.

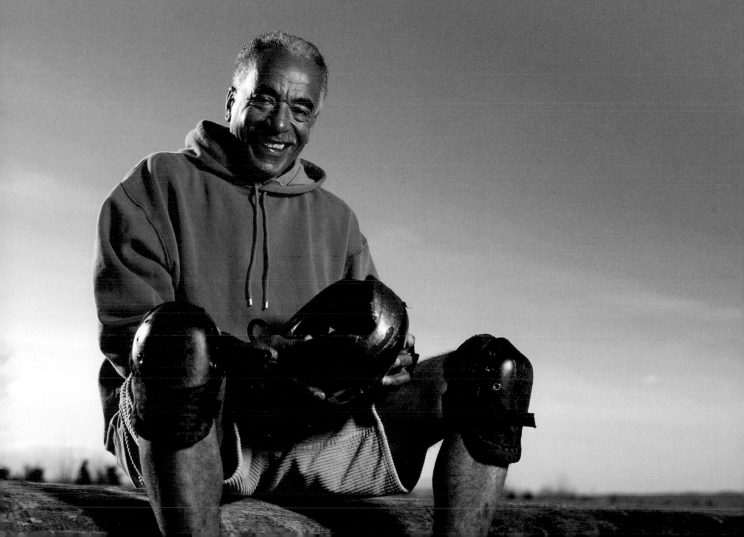

Age

The risk of gallstones increases with age. By age 70, about 35 percent of women and 20 percent of men have gallstones. One reason might be that as you get older your liver tends to secrete more cholesterol into bile.

Excess weight

Studies indicate that obese people have a much greater risk of developing gallstones than do people with a healthy weight. Excess cholesterol tends to accumulate in the bile of people who are overweight. Excess weight also decreases bile salt formation, as well as the ability of your gallbladder to contract and empty.

Diet and dieting

A diet high in fat and sugar, combined with lack of exercise and activity, increases your risk of gallstones. Fasting and rapid-weight-loss diets also increase your risk of gallstone formation because such measures alter your levels of bile salts and cholesterol and throw bile chemistry out of balance.

Some doctors prescribe the bile salt medication ursodiol (Actigall, Urso, Urso Forte) for people in rapid-weight-loss programs to offset the potential buildup of stone-forming cholesterol in bile and in the gallbladder.

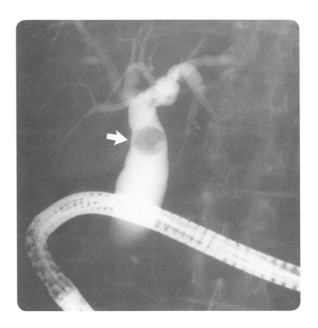

This ERCP image reveals a large gallstone (arrow) wedged in a dilated bile duct. The flexible endoscope used for the imaging test appears in the foreground.

Diagnosis

If your doctor suspects that severe, persistent abdominal pain may be caused by gallstones, you'll probably undergo one or more tests to locate the stones. They generally include an ultrasound examination and blood tests (for more details, see Chapter 4).

Ultrasound

This procedure uses sound waves to form images of your internal organs. The simple, painless examination lasts about 15 minutes. Ultrasound detects stones in your gallbladder with high accuracy but is less accurate for stones that have passed into the bile ducts.

Blood tests
Elevated levels of certain substances in your blood, including bilirubin and alkaline phosphatase, can suggest an obstruction in one of your bile ducts.

Computerized tomography
A computerized tomography (CT) scan of your abdomen can sometimes reveal gallstones that contain high levels of calcium. During a gallstone attack, your gallbladder may appear thickened on a CT or ultrasound scan.

Radionuclide scan
An imaging procedure known as a hepatobiliary iminodiacetic acid (HIDA) scan uses a radioactive tracer to track the flow of bile from your liver to your small intestine. A small amount of tracer is given to you intravenously and absorbed by the liver. The scan will show when bile infused with the tracer reaches your gallbladder.

If there's no evidence of tracer in the gallbladder, a stone may be blocking the gallbladder neck or the cystic duct, which connects to the main bile duct.

Endoscopic retrograde cholangiopancreatography
This imaging procedure, known as ERCP, allows your doctor to examine your bile ducts for blockage (see image on page 186). While you're sedated, a flexible tube with an attached camera (endoscope) is threaded through your digestive tract to the opening of the common bile duct in your duodenum. Dye injected from a catheter inside the scope enters the duct to clearly outline the biliary system on X-ray images. If a stone is discovered in one of the ducts, it usually can be removed with tools attached to the endoscope.

Treatment options

The best treatment for stones in the gallbladder, generally, is to do nothing more than watch and wait. This is often recommended if you have "silent stones," which typically don't cause signs and symptoms. Silent stones usually are discovered by accident, during diagnostic testing for other conditions.

If you've had one or more gallbladder attacks, your doctor will probably recommend surgery to remove the gallbladder, unless other health problems make surgery too risky.

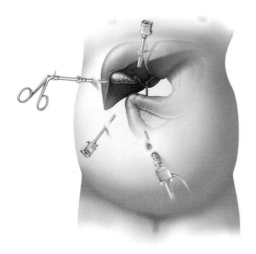

Special surgical tools are inserted through four small incisions in your abdomen during laparoscopic cholecystectomy.

Fortunately, the gallbladder is not an essential organ — it's possible for the liver to supply bile to the small intestine directly. Nonsurgical options are available but generally do not resolve the problem permanently.

Surgery

Surgery to remove the gallbladder is called a cholecystectomy (koh-luh-sis-TEK-tuh-me). It's generally safe and effective, and one of the most common surgical procedures performed in the United States.

Complete organ removal is the preferred treatment option for gallbladder attacks, simply because removing just the gallstones is often a temporary measure — new stones will form later and gallstone attacks can recur.

Rarely, surgery can be complicated by serious, hard-to-treat problems such as a torn or leaking bile duct, a blocked bile duct, bleeding, or infection.

Cholecystectomy is performed in one of two ways:

Open surgery
During this procedure, the gallbladder is removed through a large abdominal incision. Open surgery is used only occasionally today. Your doctor may recommend the procedure if your gallbladder walls are thick and hard, or there is scar tissue from earlier abdominal operations. Recovery typically involves a week's stay in the hospital, followed by about three weeks at home.

Laparoscopic surgery
The majority of gallbladder surgeries are now done laparoscopically. The Greek word *lapara* refers to the abdomen and *scope* means the use of an endoscope to guide the surgeon and to perform the tasks.

The procedure involves making several small incisions in your abdomen instead of one large one. (See the illustration on page 188.) A tube inserted through one incision injects carbon dioxide gas into the abdominal cavity, creating more space for the surgeon to see your internal organs. Instruments inserted through other incisions include an endoscope equipped with a camera for viewing the gallbladder and another equipped with a cutting device to remove the gallbladder.

Laparoscopic surgery ordinarily requires an overnight stay in the hospital. Recovery time is shorter than from open surgery because the incisions are small and the surgeon doesn't have to cut through abdominal muscles, which take longer to heal. Other advantages include less pain and less scarring.

Nonsurgical option

Your doctor may recommend nonsurgical treatment if you have complications or concerns that make surgery inadvisable. The major disadvantage of nonsurgical treatment is that the gallstones usually recur.

The primary nonsurgical option for gallstones is known as bile acid dissolution therapy. You take bile acid tablets, which dissolve cholesterol stones over several months or years. However, these tablets don't work on pigment stones or any stones that are heavily surrounded by calcium.

Ursodiol (Actigall, Urso, Urso Forte) is widely used for this therapy because it's effective and seems to have the fewest side effects, including mild diarrhea that is, for the most part, occasional. Ursodiol works best on small stones containing a large amount of

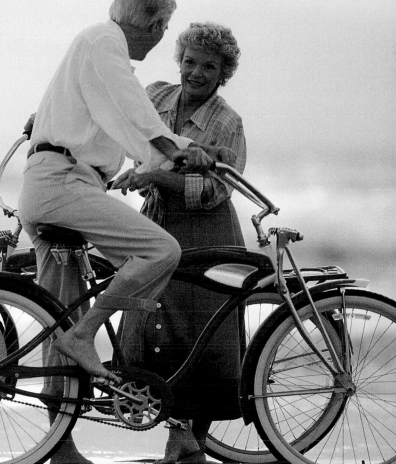

cholesterol and no detectable calcium, and when an open cystic duct allows bile to enter and exit normally.

The disadvantage of ursodiol is that its benefits are not permanent. Gallstones tend to recur in about half the people taking ursodiol within five years after they stop treatment — unless they continue the medication indefinitely.

Life without a gallbladder

Most people who have surgery to remove their gallbladders get along well without them. Your liver continues to produce enough bile to digest the fat consumed in a healthy diet. But instead of being stored in your gallbladder, bile flows out of the liver and empties directly into the small intestine.

You don't need to change eating habits after surgery. However, with bile flowing more frequently into your small intestine, you may experience a greater number of bowel movements and your stools may be softer. Many times, though, these changes are only temporary. Over time, your intestines adjust to the effects of gallbladder removal.

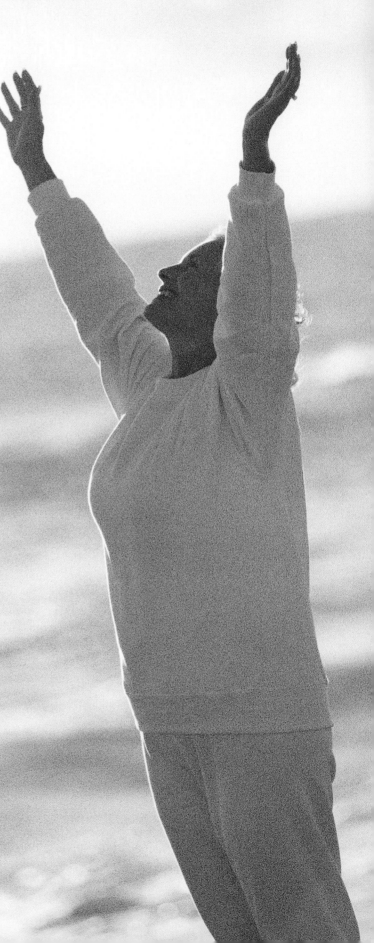

Chapter 12

Pancreatitis

It's a stomachache like you've never felt before. Severe pain that seems to bore right through your upper abdomen, from the chest to the back. You feel debilitated. Lying flat on your back causes your stomach to hurt more, but leaning forward and doubling over offers some relief. Your breathing becomes shallow because taking deep breaths causes even more pain.

These signs and symptoms are typical of pancreatitis (pan-kre-uh-TI-tis), an inflammation of the pancreas. There are two forms of this disease. The pain of acute pancreatitis is often sudden, severe and steady, and lasts for days. In contrast, chronic pancreatitis occurs in intermittent episodes and the pain typically builds up gradually. The chronic form can occur over many years.

Key signs and symptoms

- Abdominal pain
- Nausea and vomiting
- Fever
- Bloating and gas
- Foul-smelling, loose, oily stools
- Weight loss

The pancreas is an important part of your digestive system, but few people know much about its function. The organ is a long, flat gland tucked behind your stomach. The pancreatic duct connects the pancreas to the common bile duct leaving your gallbladder. The combined duct empties

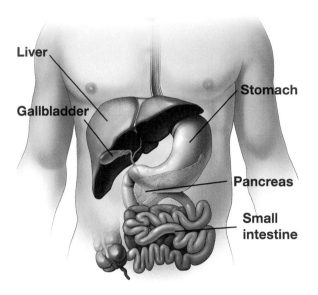

Liver

Gallbladder

Stomach

Pancreas

Small intestine

into the upper section of the small intestine (duodenum). The pancreas has two main functions:

- Produces digestive juices and enzymes that help break down fats, carbohydrates and proteins in your small intestine.

- Secretes the hormones insulin and glucagon into your bloodstream, along with somatostatin, another hormone that helps control their function. The primary role of these hormones is to regulate how your body metabolizes sugar (glucose).

Inflammation in the pancreas disrupts these functions. Most cases of pancreatitis are mild to moderate but for some people can be severe.

Acute vs. chronic

Each year, thousands of cases of acute pancreatitis are diagnosed in the United States. The main symptom is steady pain in your upper abdomen that springs up suddenly and may range from mild to severe. The pain often radiates to your back and chest and usually persists for many hours or days without relief.

The cause of acute pancreatitis is digestive enzymes that your body activates too soon. Normally, the enzymes produced in your pancreas start out in an inactive form. Only after they're transported through the pancreatic duct and into the duodenum do they become active in the digestive process. If these enzymes become activated while still in the pancreas, they irritate and inflame the gland, sometimes destroying delicate pancreatic tissues.

Eating food or drinking alcohol may make your symptoms worse. Many people with acute pancreatitis sit up and bend forward or curl up in a fetal position because these positions seem to relieve the pain.

People with severe inflammation often feel and look extremely sick. They frequently experience nausea and vomiting.

Other signs and symptoms may include a high fever, difficulty breathing and abdominal swelling (distention). The pain may become so severe that hospitalization is necessary.

Chronic pancreatitis differs from acute pancreatitis in that the inflammation is ongoing, often over many years. The chronic condition can be more difficult to diagnose because the damage occurs slowly and it may take awhile before the signs and symptoms appear. In the early stages of chronic pancreatitis, you may experience mild to severe episodes similar to acute pancreatitis.

While a few people with chronic pancreatitis experience no pain, most have intermittent periods of mild to moderate abdominal pain. The pain may be sharp and last for a few hours, or it may be a continuously dull ache that lasts for weeks.

In addition to pain, you may have nausea and vomiting, fever, bloating and gas. Eating food or drinking alcohol can make symptoms worse.

Acute pancreatitis often resolves spontaneously without long-term complications, often within a week or less. The chronic form usually causes permanent damage to the pancreas.

As inflammation persists, it slowly destroys tissue in the pancreas. The gland becomes less able to produce enzymes and hormones necessary for digestion.

An insufficient supply of digestive enzymes and hormones leads to the poor absorption of nutrients, particularly fat. This causes weight loss and the passage of fat-containing stools that are loose, foul-smelling and oily in appearance. Eventually, your cells that produce insulin are impaired, causing diabetes. Malabsorption and diabetes often don't appear until much of the gland has been destroyed.

Primary causes

Acute pancreatitis can occur for various reasons but, in some cases, its cause remains unknown. The two most common causes are gallstones and excessive alcohol use.

Gallstones

Many people with acute pancreatitis also have gallstones. Sometimes these stones migrate out of the gallbladder and move through the common bile duct. The stones may become lodged at

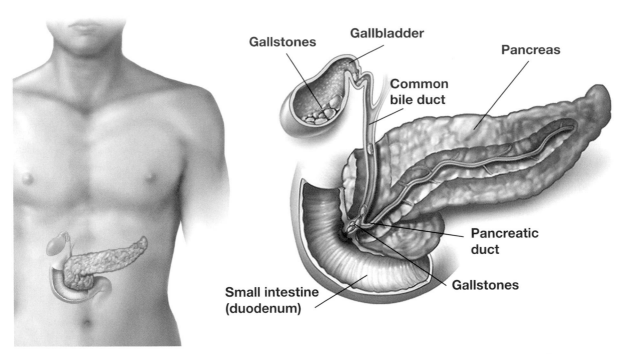

Gallstones that leave the gallbladder and block the pancreatic duct are a common cause of acute pancreatitis. Digestive juices produced by the pancreas are trapped, inflaming delicate tissues.

the junction with the pancreatic duct, near the entrance to the duodenum, blocking the flow of pancreatic juices into the digestive tract. This blockage causes a backflow into the pancreas. Digestive enzymes that typically are inactive until they reach the duodenum may now be activated while still in the pancreas. This activation produces inflammation, causing signs and symptoms associated with pancreatitis.

Usually this duct blockage is temporary, and the stones eventually pass into the duodenum. Gallstones do not cause chronic pancreatitis.

Alcohol

Heavy alcohol use over many years is a leading cause of pancreatitis. A recent study suggests five or more alcoholic drinks a day may establish for threshold for chronic pancreatitis.

It's unclear how alcohol damages the pancreas. One theory holds that excessive alcohol leads to the formation of protein plugs — precursors to small stones — that build up in the pancreas and block parts of the pancreatic duct. Another theory is that alcohol directly injures pancreatic tissue.

Less common causes

A number of other factors have been identified that may lead to either the acute or chronic forms of pancreatitis. These factors include:

- Structural abnormalities of the pancreas or abdominal trauma
- Following major abdominal surgery or certain invasive diagnostic tests such as endoscopic retrograde cholangiopancreatography (ERCP)
- Blockage from calcium deposits or stones in the pancreatic duct or common bile duct
- Family history of pancreatitis
- High levels of triglycerides (hypertriglyceridemia) or of calcium in the blood (hypercalcemia)
- Cystic fibrosis
- Cigarette smoking, especially if you also drink alcohol
- Bacterial or viral infection
- Certain medications, including blood pressure lowering drugs in the thiazide diuretic class, antibiotics such as tetracyclines and sulfonamides, and some drugs that treat cancer and autoimmune diseases

Occasionally, a complication of acute pancreatitis will lead to chronic pancreatitis. Sometimes, young adults with cystic fibrosis and associated gene abnormalities have episodes of acute pancreatitis that eventually develop into chronic pancreatitis.

Some people are also born with a hereditary form of pancreatitis that can cause acute attacks during childhood or adolescence, but eventually develops into chronic pancreatitis.

Although many possible causes for pancreatitis have been identified, there are a surprising number of individuals for whom no cause is apparent. Perhaps closer inspection might clarify these cases. Researchers suspect that some acute attacks may be linked to gallstones that are too small to detect or identify. Other attacks may involve unidentified genetic mutations.

Treating acute pancreatitis

Diagnosing pancreatitis can be difficult, and several tests may be necessary to help pinpoint the problem. If your doctor suspects acute pancreatitis, he or she will check your abdomen for pain and tenderness. A sample of your blood may be analyzed for abnormalities that signal acute inflammation, such as:

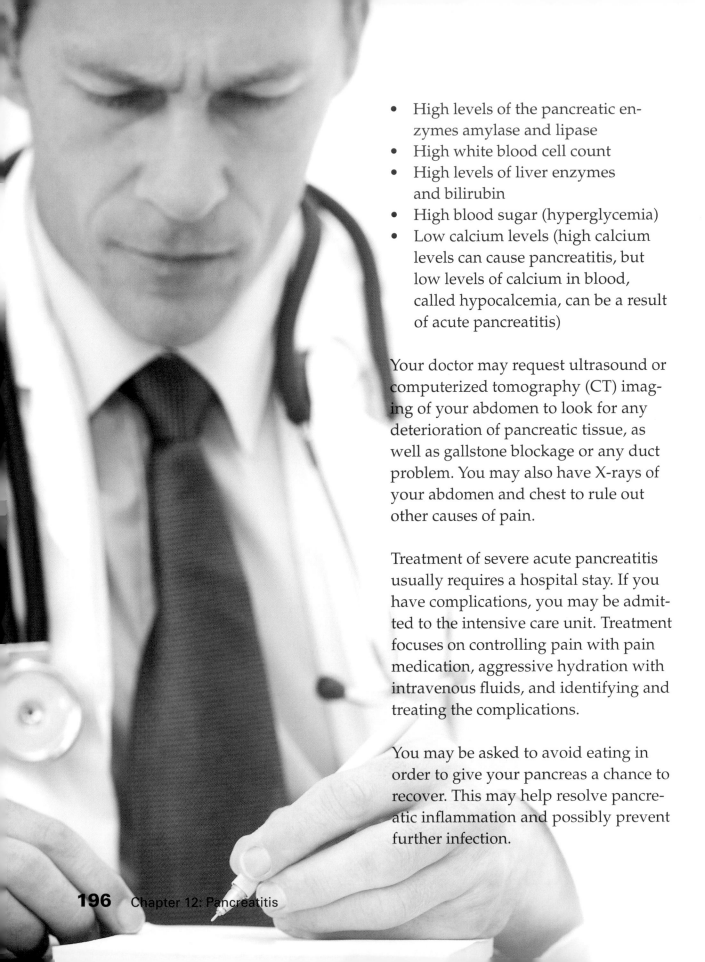

- High levels of the pancreatic enzymes amylase and lipase
- High white blood cell count
- High levels of liver enzymes and bilirubin
- High blood sugar (hyperglycemia)
- Low calcium levels (high calcium levels can cause pancreatitis, but low levels of calcium in blood, called hypocalcemia, can be a result of acute pancreatitis)

Your doctor may request ultrasound or computerized tomography (CT) imaging of your abdomen to look for any deterioration of pancreatic tissue, as well as gallstone blockage or any duct problem. You may also have X-rays of your abdomen and chest to rule out other causes of pain.

Treatment of severe acute pancreatitis usually requires a hospital stay. If you have complications, you may be admitted to the intensive care unit. Treatment focuses on controlling pain with pain medication, aggressive hydration with intravenous fluids, and identifying and treating the complications.

You may be asked to avoid eating in order to give your pancreas a chance to recover. This may help resolve pancreatic inflammation and possibly prevent further infection.

If your attack is caused by gallstones blocking the pancreatic duct, your doctor may recommend a procedure to remove the stones. You may eventually need surgery to remove the gallbladder if gallstones continue to pose problems. If alcohol is the cause, treatment may include therapy to stop drinking. However, complete abstinence from alcohol doesn't guarantee you won't have another attack.

Mild cases of acute pancreatitis generally improve in three to seven days. Moderate to severe cases may take longer to resolve. Once the inflammation is under control, you may begin drinking clear liquids and eating bland foods again. With time, you can go back to your normal diet.

Complications of acute pancreatitis

Acute pancreatitis may lead to destruction of part of the pancreas (pancreatic necrosis), inflammation and fluid buildup in and around the gland, and failure of other organs, including the heart, lungs and kidneys.

Infection
A damaged pancreas may become infected with bacteria that have spread from the small intestine. Signs of infection include fever, chills, elevated white blood cell count and organ failure.

A radiologist may extract a fluid sample from the pancreas, which can be tested for bacterial infection. If the tests are positive, you'll receive antibiotics. Some people also need surgery or endoscopic- or radiologic-guided procedures to drain or remove infected areas. Sometimes, multiple procedures are necessary.

Pseudocysts
Cyst-like, fluid-filled blisters called pseudocysts may form on the pancreas or extend from the gland after an attack of acute pancreatitis. If the cyst is small, no special treatment is necessary. If it is large and becomes infected or causes bleeding, intervention is necessary. Your doctor may drain the cyst through an endoscopic- or radiologic-guided catheter, or you may need surgery to remove the cyst.

Abscess
A collection of pus, or abscess, can develop near the pancreas about three to four weeks after the onset of acute pancreatitis. Treatment involves draining the abscess with a catheter guided by an endoscope or with radiologic imaging, or with a surgical procedure.

Treating chronic pancreatitis

The periods of abdominal pain that often appear with chronic pancreatitis may be confused initially with acute pancreatitis. But you may also start to lose weight without trying, and your stools may be oily and foul-smelling.

To confirm a diagnosis of chronic pancreatitis, your doctor will likely take samples of blood and stool. Blood tests can identify abnormalities associated with chronic pancreatitis and help rule out acute inflammation. The stool test measures fat content in your feces. Excess fat occurs in stool when it isn't absorbed in your small intestine.

Your doctor may have you undergo X-ray, ultrasound or endoscopic procedures to look for evidence of a blockage in the pancreatic duct or common bile duct. You may also need additional tests if your doctor is concerned about the possibility of other diseases, such as pancreatic cancer. Having chronic pancreatitis puts you at a slightly higher risk of pancreatic cancer.

The main goals of treatment for chronic pancreatitis are to control pain and treat malabsorption problems.

Relieving pain

Unlike acute pancreatitis, in which pain often disappears within a few days to weeks, pain lingers with chronic pancreatitis. In fact, persistent pain may be the greatest challenge of treating this chronic condition.

Your doctor may prescribe supplements containing pancreatic enzymes, in addition to conventional pain relievers. It's believed that this therapy works by increasing the levels of digestive enzymes active in your duodenum. This, in turn, decreases demand for the secretion of enzymes from the pancreas, which reduces pressure, and hence, pain, within the pancreas.

For severe pain that can't be controlled, treatment options include surgery to remove damaged tissue or procedures to block pain signals or deaden those nerves transmitting the pain.

Malabsorption therapy

Enzyme supplements containing pancrelipase (Creon, Pancreaze) can help treat malabsorption — absorption problems during digestion — caused by pancreatitis. The tablets replace enzymes no longer produced by the pancreas, helping to restore normal digestion. They also assist fat absorption that is otherwise lost in your stool.

Depending on how the enzyme supplements are prepared, you may take up to eight tablets with meals — two tablets after a few bites of food, four tablets during the meal, and two tablets toward the end. Supplements should also be taken with snacks.

Treating diabetes

Chronic pancreatitis may cause diabetes. Treatment is similar to that of type 2 diabetes and usually involves maintaining a healthy diet and getting regular exercise. Some people also need insulin injections. Your doctor can explain how to manage the condition and prevent complications.

Managing chronic pancreatitis

People with chronic pancreatitis often experience signs and symptoms throughout their lives. People with acute pancreatitis, on the other hand, often recover completely.

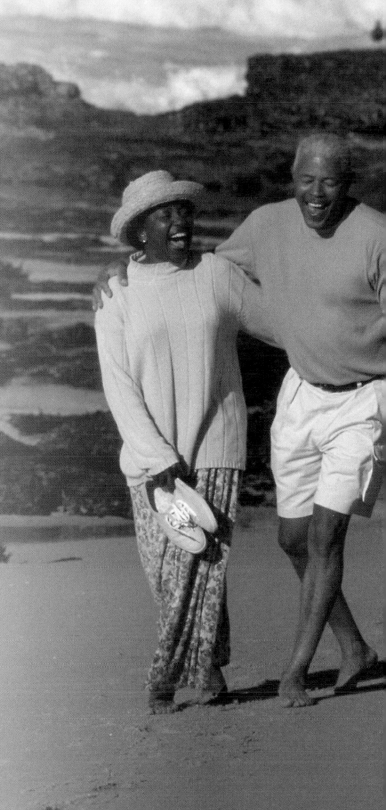

Even if you experience no lingering signs and symptoms, it's important to keep your pancreas healthy:

Avoid alcohol

If you can't voluntarily stop drinking alcohol, get treatment for alcoholism. Abstaining from alcohol may not reduce the pain, but it will reduce your risk of dying of your disease.

Stop smoking

Smoking has several bad effects for people with pancreatitis. It reduces pancreatic function, hastens the development of stones that block the pancreatic duct and increases the risk of pancreatic cancer.

Eat smaller meals

The more food you eat during a meal, the greater the amount of digestive juices your pancreas must produce. Instead of large meals, eat smaller, more frequent meals.

Find safe ways to control pain

Talk with your doctor about options for controlling pain, including the benefits and risks of prescription and over-the-counter pain relievers. Although often effective, these medications carry the risk of side effects, including drug dependence and stomach problems.

Chapter 13

Liver disease

The liver is your largest single internal organ and possibly the most complex. It may also be one of the most underappreciated. The organ has a triangular shape, consisting of two main lobes. Its specialized cells are connected by the biliary system — an intricate system of bile ducts and blood vessels.

The liver is hardworking and multitasking, playing critical roles in your body's metabolic, digestive and regulatory systems, but it goes about its work without drawing much attention to itself. For that reason, it's easy to ignore the liver until something goes wrong.

Due to its complexity and frequent exposure to many potentially harmful substances, the liver is vulnerable to infection, inflammation and blockage.

There are more than 100 liver diseases and conditions, and damage that occurs to the organ can be hard to reverse.

Your liver is capable of performing many complicated tasks simultaneously that are essential to the proper functioning of your body. These tasks include:

Processing food into energy
The liver processes most of the nutrients absorbed from your intestines. It converts many nutrients into forms that can be used by your body (metabolized), and stores other nutrients, such as vitamin A and iron, for later use. The liver also manufactures cholesterol, blood-clotting factors, specific proteins such as albumin, and bile, a fluid that's essential for the digestion of fat.

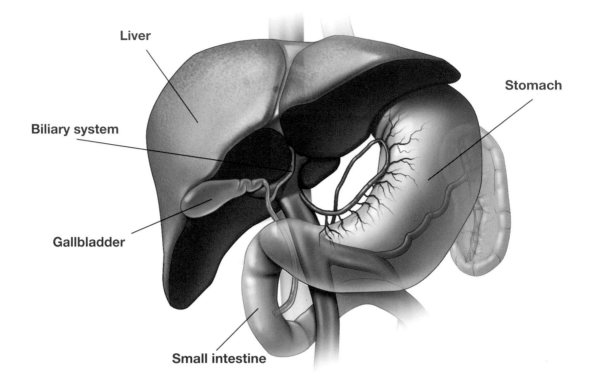

Liver

Stomach

Biliary system

Gallbladder

Small intestine

Detoxifying your body

The liver filters waste from your blood. It converts some potentially harmful substances, drugs and toxins into forms that are less harmful and can be removed from your body via bile and, subsequently, stool.

Regulating composition of blood

The liver regulates the composition of your blood, in particular, the amounts of sugar (glucose), protein and fat that enter your bloodstream. The liver also removes a substance called bilirubin from your blood, which is a byproduct from the breakdown of red blood cells.

It's common for people to not associate digestive problems with the liver. However, signs and symptoms such as lack of appetite, weight loss and nausea actually may stem from a liver disorder rather than the stomach or intestinal problem you thought you had.

Liver problems include a wide range of diseases and conditions that damage liver tissue or function. They may be caused by infection, trauma or exposure to toxins. They may be a result of inflammation or scarring. If your liver isn't functioning properly, your body may not be getting the nutrients it needs, leading to weight loss and fatigue. A buildup of waste and toxins in your blood can cause yellowing of your skin and eyes (jaundice), loss of appetite, nausea and, sometimes, vomiting. Swelling of the ankles, fluid accumulation in the abdominal cavity (ascites), bruising and confusion (hepatic encephalopathy) also may occur.

Hepatitis

The most common liver disease is hepatitis, an inflammation of the liver. If an organ becomes inflamed, it's trying to fight infection or heal an injury. In addition to pain and swelling, inflammation disrupts your liver's ability to filter harmful substances from your body.

When that happens, waste products such as bilirubin build up in your bloodstream, causing your skin and eyes to turn yellow (jaundice). If the inflammation continues unchecked, your liver may be permanently damaged. There are several forms of hepatitis.

Alcohol- or drug-induced hepatitis
The most common form of hepatitis occurs in people who drink excessive amounts of alcohol or who take certain medications. Inflammation stems from

Hepatitis
Key signs and symptoms

- Fatigue
- Loss of appetite
- Nausea
- Unexplained weight loss
- Yellowing of skin and eyes (jaundice)

the toxic chemicals that your body produces as it breaks down the alcohol or drugs. Over time, these chemicals damage liver cells and interfere with your liver's ability to do its job.

Just how alcohol damages the liver, and why it does so, isn't entirely clear. Perhaps one-third of heavy drinkers get alcoholic hepatitis, but the condition may often go undiagnosed. Women generally develop alcoholic hepatitis more quickly than men do, and in women, smaller amounts of alcohol are generally involved.

Medications that most commonly lead to drug-induced hepatitis are nonprescription pain relievers, especially if the drugs are taken frequently or combined with alcohol. Nonprescription pain relievers include aspirin, acetaminophen (Tylenol, others) and nonsteroidal anti-inflammatory drugs (NSAIDs), such as ibuprofen (Advil, Motrin, others), naproxen (Aleve) and ketoprofen.

Although in most people, the following prescription medications don't cause any problems, in people with liver disease, they may be damaging:

- Certain high blood pressure medications, including calcium channel blockers and angiotensin-converting enzyme (ACE) inhibitors
- Certain antibiotics, including tuberculosis drugs such as isoniazid
- Valproic acid, an anti-seizure medication
- Methotrexate, a cancer medication also used to treat psoriasis
- Some diabetes medications

Hepatitis A
This highly contagious form of hepatitis is spread by food or water contaminated by the feces of someone who has the hepatitis A virus, or by close contact with another person already infected with the disease. This is the form of hepatitis that you'll most likely encounter during international travel. It's estimated that about 1 in 3 Americans has evidence of a past infection.

Outbreaks of hepatitis A have been traced to raw shellfish, strawberries, green onions, and other food and produce that may have been contaminated by irrigation water or by an infected worker who failed to wash his or her hands before handling the food.

Hepatitis A usually resolves itself without treatment. In a few cases, especially in adults older than 40, it may cause severe symptoms requiring medical treatment and perhaps hospitalization. In rare cases, the condition can be fatal. Practicing good hygiene is one of the best ways to protect yourself.

Hepatitis B
This hepatitis virus, also highly contagious, is found in blood and semen, and commonly transmitted through unprotected sexual contact or by sharing contaminated syringes and needles during intravenous drug use. At greatest risk are people with multiple sexual partners, users of illicit drugs and hospital workers exposed to blood.

At birth, a newborn can be infected with hepatitis B if the mother is already infected. However, some people are infected without any known risk factor. Hepatitis B is not spread through hugging, sneezing, coughing, consuming food or water, or sharing eating and drinking utensils.

An estimated 800,000 to 1.4 million Americans may have a chronic hepatitis B infection. Worldwide, about 350 million people are carriers of the virus. The disease is more common in some parts of the world — for example, Asia and sub-Saharan Africa — than in other parts, such as North America.

Hepatitis C

Hepatitis C is the most common cause of viral hepatitis in the United States. It is spread through blood and blood products and contaminated needles. Users of illicit drugs who share paraphernalia account for many of the new infections. Contrary to popular myth, hepatitis C isn't spread through breastfeeding, hugging, sneezing, coughing, consuming food or water, or sharing eating and drinking utensils. Unlike hepatitis B, it's unlikely to spread via sexual intercourse.

People who received blood transfusions before 1992 also are at increased risk of hepatitis C. In 1992, blood banks began screening for the virus. Because this form of hepatitis can take decades to progress, it's unclear how many of the people who had blood transfusions before 1992 may be infected.

Screening for hepatitis C

A simple screening test can pinpoint hepatitis C antibodies in blood, often identifying the disease before signs and symptoms develop and serious liver damage occurs. Have a screening test if you:

- Are using or have used illicit intravenous or intranasal drugs (even once)
- Received a blood transfusion before 1992
- Received a transplanted organ before 1992
- Received blood-clotting factor before 1987
- Have been accidentally exposed to the blood of others
- Are undergoing hemodialysis (or have undergone the procedure)
- Have hemophilia
- Have had sexual relations or have shared razors, toothbrushes or nail clippers with someone who has hepatitis C
- Have had unprotected sex with multiple partners

In the United States, approximately 3.2 million people are chronically infected with hepatitis C. Many develop scarring (cirrhosis) of the liver. Hepatitis C is also the leading reason for liver transplants in adults. Each year, 10,000 to 12,000 people die of liver failure stemming from the disease.

Hepatitis D
To get this bloodborne virus, you must already have hepatitis B. Hepatitis D survives by attaching itself to the hepatitis B virus. Hepatitis D is not common in the United States.

Hepatitis E
Most cases reported in the United States of this foodborne virus involve travelers to parts of the world where the disease is prevalent, such as the Middle East, Asia, Mexico and South America. Pregnant women are at high risk of death if they get hepatitis E.

Autoimmune hepatitis
This form of hepatitis is much more common among women than men. The disease is believed to be caused by an agent that triggers your immune system to attack liver cells.

Nonalcoholic fatty liver disease
This condition, commonly known as NAFLD, describes the accumulation of excess fat in the liver — similar to what happens in alcohol-induced hepatitis — but an individual with NAFLD drinks little or no alcohol.

The condition most often occurs in people who are obese or who have diabetes or high triglyceride levels. For most people, NAFLD causes no signs and symptoms and no complications develop. But in some people with fatty liver disease, the fat deposits can cause inflammation and permanent scarring of the liver.

Acute vs. chronic forms

There can be a wide range of time in how long hepatitis signs and symptoms last. They may persist for only a short time and then disappear (acute hepatitis), or they may continue for the rest of your life (chronic hepatitis).

Acute hepatitis
Acute hepatitis generally causes little or no permanent liver damage. The attack may develop suddenly or gradually, but usually subsides within six months or less. As your body's defenses overcome the virus or drug and clear it from your body, the liver inflammation and associated signs and symptoms subside and then disappear.

Hepatitis A and E are acute forms of the condition that do not become chronic. Hepatitis B also is acute, but in some cases the inflammation can become chronic. Newborns exposed to hepatitis B usually develop a chronic disease.

Chronic hepatitis

Chronic hepatitis is generally considered to be hepatitis that lasts for more than six months. The liver remains inflamed, even if you may not show any signs and symptoms. Some people live with hepatitis for more than 20 years without even realizing they have the condition. Over time, inflammation causes scar tissue to form in the liver (cirrhosis), eventually leading to liver failure. People with cirrhosis also are at increased risk of liver cancer.

Most cases of hepatitis C turn into the chronic form, even though the condition often starts as an acute infection. Hepatitis C accounts for between 60 and 70 percent of all chronic cases of viral hepatitis, and up to 50 percent of cirrhosis, end-stage liver disease and liver cancer.

Chronic hepatitis can develop along different paths. It may progress slowly and damage only a limited portion of your liver, or it may progress rapidly, causing extensive liver damage.

Diagnosing hepatitis

Because the signs and symptoms of hepatitis often differ from one person to the next, there aren't common warning signs of the disease. For some people, fatigue and yellowing of the skin and eyes (jaundice) are early indicators.

If the doctor suspects hepatitis, you'll likely need to respond to a series of questions regarding your health and lifestyle. Did you have a blood transfusion before 1992? Have you recently visited a foreign country? Do you practice unsafe sex? Have you used self-injected illicit drugs?

A physical examination is typically the next step in diagnosis. Your doctor will feel (palpate) your upper abdomen for evidence of an enlarged, shrunken or hardened liver. He or she will also look for other signs and symptoms of liver disease, such as swelling of the abdomen, legs and ankles, and jaundice.

In addition, you'll likely have tests that can measure certain enzymes or proteins in your blood. (In people who don't exhibit signs and symptoms, a routine blood donation or a blood test for another condition is often the way the disease is first detected.) Blood tests for liver disease, called liver tests or liver function tests, can identify four types of abnormalities:

Liver cell damage

If liver cells are inflamed or damaged, the enzymes normally found in those cells will leak into the bloodstream and show up in test results. Two tests that check for elevated enzyme levels are the alanine aminotransferase (ALT) and aspartate aminotransferase (AST) tests.

Reduced liver function

When your liver is impaired, usually because of severe injury, it's not able to produce protein (albumin) as it normally does, or provide certain blood-clotting factors (prothrombin). Albumin level and prothrombin time tests measure these functions.

High levels of alkaline phosphatase

This enzyme is produced primarily by cells located in small bile ducts in your liver. The levels may increase with conditions that affect the ducts or liver.

Increased bilirubin

Bilirubin is a substance produced by the normal breakdown of red blood cells. If your liver isn't removing bilirubin, this test measures elevated levels that circulate in your bloodstream. Certain blood diseases also can increase bilirubin levels in blood.

Blood tests often provide clear enough indication of hepatitis to make a diagnosis. However, your doctor may remove a sample of liver tissue (biopsy) for laboratory examination. These samples can help identify the specific type of hepatitis you have. They may also indicate how severe the inflammation is and whether there is any permanent liver damage.

Treating hepatitis

Treatment options for hepatitis will depend on the form of the disease you have. For hepatitis A or E, you probably won't need any medication. However, you may require hospitalization if you're pregnant, dehydrated or an older adult, or if you have other health problems. In rare cases when hepatitis A leads to liver failure, a liver transplant may be considered.

Treatment for other forms of hepatitis, including B, C and D, is still evolving. The primary goals are to relieve signs and symptoms and to prevent scarring (cirrhosis) of the liver. For the viral forms of hepatitis, another goal is to reduce or eliminate the amount of virus present in your body fluids (viral levels). Treatment may involve one or more of the following approaches:

Corticosteroids

Corticosteroids reduce liver inflammation by suppressing the immune system. These drugs are used to treat chronic autoimmune hepatitis, providing short-term relief of signs and symptoms in most people. However, many individuals experience a relapse within six months of stopping the medication.

Corticosteroids aren't prescribed for viral forms of hepatitis because suppressing the immune system may encourage the virus to multiply rapidly.

The two most commonly used corticosteroids are prednisone and prednisolone. Side effects may include weight gain, skin problems, elevated blood pressure, diabetes, cataracts, infection, osteoporosis and a moon-shaped face.

Once the disease is in remission, your doctor may gradually reduce dosage to the lowest possible level to avoid or lessen side effects. Other immunosuppressant drugs, such as azathioprine (Azasan, Imuran) and mercaptopurine (Purinethol), also may help reduce the amount of corticosteroids taken.

Interferons

Interferons are naturally occurring proteins in your body that inhibit viruses from replicating. People with hepatitis B or C aren't able to produce enough interferons to ward off the virus, so synthetic forms may be injected to boost their interferon levels.

Currently, the treatment showing most promise for hepatitis C is a form of interferon (pegylated), given by injection, that's combined with the drug ribavirin (Rebetol, Ribasphere), which is taken orally. Available interferon drugs are peginterferon alfa-2b (Peg-Intron) and peginterferon alfa-2a (Pegasys). This combination treatment is usually prescribed for either 24 weeks or 48 weeks.

Because of its side effects, interferon isn't recommended for people with a history of major depression, low blood cell counts or autoimmune disease, or who abuse alcohol or drugs. Side effects include flu-like symptoms, fatigue, depression, and reduced white blood cell and blood platelet counts. Ribavirin has been associated with anemia. Neither medication can be given to a woman or to her partner during pregnancy.

Other antiviral medications

Various medications, which function in similar fashion as interferons, can interfere with the ability of the hepatitis virus to replicate. These drugs are often used to treat individuals with chronic hepatitis B. (Pegylated interferon may also be used.) The drugs, all taken in tablet form once a day, have minimal side effects and seem to be well tolerated by most people. However, signs and symptoms may worsen severely when you stop taking the drugs. The antiviral drugs include:

- Adefovir dipivoxil (Hepsera)
- Entecavir (Baraclude)
- Lamivudine (Epivir-HBV)
- Telbivudine (Tyzeka)
- Tenofovir (Viread)

Liver transplantation

When liver damage is extensive and medications are no longer helpful, your doctor may discuss the possibility of a liver transplant. You cannot live without a functioning liver, and transplantation may be your best option. Many people lead normal lives following the procedure. Unfortunately, the number of people awaiting transplants far exceeds the number of donated organs.

Furthermore, transplantation does not necessarily cure the disease. If you have hepatitis C or B, there's a chance that the hepatitis virus will recur in a new liver. Liver transplant recipients with hepatitis B routinely receive immunoglobulin injections and medications to reduce the risk of recurrence.

Living with hepatitis

Once you have hepatitis, your risk of getting another form of the virus has increased. Therefore, it's important to stay healthy and avoid exposure to additional risks. What you can do in terms of self-care varies, but the following generally applies to everyone:

Rest

If you have acute hepatitis, get adequate rest, drink plenty of fluids and eat a healthy, high-calorie diet. This strengthens your immune system to fight off the virus.

Avoid alcohol

Alcohol can aggravate inflammation and speed the progression of liver disease to cirrhosis and organ failure.

Use medications carefully

Many medications impair liver function, especially if taken regularly. If your liver isn't working properly, it has trouble removing toxins produced by the drugs. Your doctor should be aware of any medication you're taking, including over-the-counter drugs.

Maintain a healthy lifestyle

A healthy lifestyle includes eating a balanced, nutritious diet and getting adequate exercise. In addition to improving your physical health, good nutrition and exercise can help overcome depression, a common problem for people with hepatitis.

Preventing hepatitis

The following precautions may help you avoid viral forms of hepatitis.

Immunization
There are effective vaccines for preventing hepatitis A and B. Depending on the type of vaccine used, you may require two or three injections. Since hepatitis A is a risk when traveling to most parts of the world, consult your doctor regarding a hepatitis A vaccine before you travel.

Almost anyone can receive the vaccine for hepatitis B, including infants, older adults and those with compromised immune systems. Children born to mothers infected with hepatitis B can be vaccinated soon after birth.

Food preparation
Since hepatitis A and E can spread through contaminated food and drink, follow these safe-food-handling habits:

- Thoroughly wash all fruits and vegetables.

- Cook foods thoroughly — freezing doesn't kill a virus.
- When visiting developing countries, use only bottled water for drinking, cooking and brushing your teeth, or tap water that's been boiled for at least 10 minutes.

Workplace precaution
In health care settings, follow all infection control procedures, including washing hands and wearing gloves. In child-care settings, which are high-risk areas for hepatitis A infections, wash your hands thoroughly after changing or handling diapers.

Other precautions
Also practice these good health habits to reduce your risk of hepatitis:

- If you have sexual relations with multiple partners — a risk factor for hepatitis B and C — use a latex condom with each sexual contact.
- Don't share drug syringes.
- If you undergo acupuncture, make sure the needles are sterilized.
- Avoid body piercing and tattooing unless you can be sure the instruments and dyes are safe (dedicated to one person only).
- Don't share toothbrushes, razors, nail clippers or other items that may come into contact with blood.

Hemochromatosis

Hemochromatosis is an inherited abnormality that causes your intestines to absorb too much iron from the food you eat, leading to iron overload. The extra iron enters your bloodstream and is stored in certain organs, primarily in the liver, heart and pancreas.

Although you carry the genetic condition from birth, signs and symptoms generally don't appear until midlife — usually between ages 30 and 50 in men, and after age 50 in women. Some people never exhibit signs and symptoms. For others, the few early signs and symptoms mimic those of other common conditions, making it difficult to diagnose the condition.

Left untreated, hemochromatosis can lead to organ damage, particularly to the heart and liver, and in the reproductive system. It can damage joints, increase your risk of diabetes and cause darkening of your skin (sometimes called bronze diabetes).

The good news is that unlike the various forms of hepatitis, hemochromatosis is easily treated. If the condition is discovered early, permanent damage can usually be prevented.

Hemochromatosis Key signs and symptoms

- Chronic fatigue
- Joint pain
- Loss of sex drive (libido) or impotence
- Infertility
- Hypothyroidism

A genetic flaw

In rare cases, iron overload may stem from repeated blood transfusions. But by far the most common cause of the disease is a mutation in a gene — the HFE gene, discovered in 1996 — that helps control the amount of iron that your small intestine absorbs.

You inherit one HFE gene from each of your parents. If both parents pass mutated HFE genes to you, you may develop hemochromatosis — you won't have the condition with only one mutated gene. Factors that increase your risk of hereditary hemochromatosis include being male, being of Northern European descent, and having a first-degree relative — a parent or sibling — who also has the condition.

Diagnosing the problem

At any stage, even before signs and symptoms appear, your doctor can detect iron overload with blood tests. A serum transferrin saturation test measures the amount of iron in your blood. A serum ferritin test measures how much iron is stored in your liver. Because other conditions can cause elevated test results, both tests are needed to diagnose hemochromatosis. A genetic test can confirm that you're carrying two abnormal copies of the HFE gene. A biopsy can determine the extent of the damage to your liver.

Many people live with high iron levels for years, and the liver may be damaged by the time their condition is diagnosed. The average time from onset of signs and symptoms to diagnosis is about 10 years. This disorder often goes undiagnosed in premenopausal women because they lose blood each month through menstruation, and also via pregnancy. Their iron levels decrease, delaying signs and symptoms.

Should you be screened?

Some but not all experts recommend that adults have a transferrin saturation test at least once during their lifetimes — preferably in early adulthood — to measure the iron level in their blood. Nearly all experts recommend checking for iron overload if there's a family history of hemochromatosis or signs and symptoms of the condition. Screening for hemochromatosis isn't usually included in routine blood tests.

Experts don't recommend genetic screening of all adults because the test is expensive and not everyone with this genetic defect has iron overload. However, if you have a close blood relative with hemochromatosis, such as a brother, sister, child or parent, you may benefit from having a genetic test to see if you're at risk. If you do carry two abnormal copies of the HFE gene but complications haven't yet developed from the disease, you and your doctor can take steps to prevent future problems.

Other inherited liver diseases

Wilson's disease. With this condition, your body accumulates excessive amounts of copper, leading to organ damage. Like hemochromatosis, Wilson's disease stems from a flawed gene. Nearly everyone with the disease has signs and symptoms by age 40, which may include liver tenderness, weight loss, fatigue, mild jaundice, and neurological or psychiatric problems. If caught early, Wilson's disease is treatable with medications that remove excess copper from your body.

Alpha-1-antitrypsin deficiency. This disorder results from a genetic defect that causes your body to produce abnormal forms of the alpha-1-antitrypsin protein, an enzyme inhibitor that helps protect your lungs. A deficiency of this protein may lead to lung and liver disease, although most people with alpha-1-antitrypsin deficiency don't develop serious liver disease.

Gilbert syndrome. This mild disorder is quite common and doesn't lead to liver damage, but jaundice may develop periodically, especially following prolonged fasting or infections such as colds or the flu.

Treatment to remove iron

Doctors can treat hemochromatosis safely and effectively by regularly removing blood from your body (phlebotomy). The goal is to reduce iron levels to normal. The amount of blood drawn depends on your age, overall health and degree of iron overload.

Once or twice a week, a pint of blood is withdrawn from a vein in your arm, in the same way as you make a blood donation. Your body normally contains 1.5 to 2 grams of stored iron. People with hemochromatosis can have up to 40 grams. Each pint of blood removed contains about 250 milligrams of iron, so it may take several months to a few years to remove all of the excess iron.

After reaching a normal iron level, most people continue to need blood removed three to four times a year to keep iron from building up. If the disease has damaged your liver or other organs, you may need other treatments.

Reducing iron in your diet

It's not necessary or advisable to remove all iron from your diet, but you want to avoid consuming excessive amounts of the mineral. Products to be avoided include iron supplements and multivitamins with iron.

You should also avoid alcohol completely and limit excessive consumption of vitamin C. Alcohol increases the risk of liver damage. Vitamin C facilitates iron absorption. Consuming excessive amounts of vitamin C may increase your iron level.

Cirrhosis

Cirrhosis is the term used to describe scarring of the liver. It occurs in response to chronic liver damage that may take place repeatedly over years. Each time your liver is injured, it tries to repair itself. In the process, scar tissue forms. With mild cirrhosis, your liver makes repairs and continues its functions. But as more and more scar tissue builds up, liver function becomes increasingly more difficult.

Most often, cirrhosis is a byproduct of chronic inflammation caused by alcohol abuse or hepatitis, including hepatitis B, hepatitis C, and autoimmune hepatitis. Cirrhosis can also result from hemochromatosis, Wilson's disease or alpha-1-antitrypsin deficiency. Other causes of cirrhosis include:

Primary biliary cirrhosis

The biliary system includes an intricate network of tiny bile ducts in the liver tissue itself. For unknown reasons, inflammation and scarring may occur in the ducts, disrupting or blocking the flow of bile. Primary biliary cirrhosis occurs far more often among women than men, generally between the ages of 30 and 60. Some people with the disease are able to live normal lives and never develop signs and symptoms.

The name *primary biliary cirrhosis* isn't entirely accurate because cirrhosis develops only in the later stages of the disease. Other complications may include inflamed joints and osteoporosis, resulting in thin bones and fractures due to the calcium loss, and sicca syndrome, a condition in which your tear glands and salivary glands fail to produce enough lubrication. Liver transplant is the only treatment that may cure the disease.

Primary sclerosing cholangitis

Cholangitis (koh-lan-JIE-tis) refers to inflammation of the bile ducts, while the term *sclerosing* (skluh-ROHS-ing) describes hardening of the ducts due to chronic inflammation. In this condition, which may stem from an autoimmune disorder, the walls of the primary bile ducts thicken and close.

Cirrhosis
Key signs
and symptoms

- Loss of appetite
- Weight loss
- Weakness and fatigue
- Abdominal swelling
- Yellowing of skin and eyes (jaundice)
- Gastrointestinal bleeding (varices)
- Sleepiness or confusion

Primary sclerosing cholangitis is a progressive disease that leads to liver damage and, eventually, liver failure. About 70 percent of people with the disease are men, and many of them also have inflammatory bowel disease. Liver transplant is the only known cure, but transplants are typically reserved for people in severe stages of liver disease.

Diagnosing cirrhosis

If signs and symptoms suggest liver disease, your doctor will feel (palpate) your upper abdomen for evidence of an enlarged, firm liver. However, as cirrhosis advances, the liver may actually shrink. The swelling of your abdomen from fluid accumulation in your peritoneal cavity (ascites) may be another warning sign of the disease.

Most often, cirrhosis is first suspected after abnormal blood tests indicate that your liver isn't functioning properly. These tests may include a complete blood count and a bilirubin test.

To determine the cause and extent of the disease, your doctor may want to evaluate images of your liver produced with ultrasound, computerized tomography (CT) or magnetic resonance imaging (MRI). In addition, a biopsy may be taken to help determine the extent of liver damage. Ultrasound and MRI also can detect stiffness or lack of elasticity in your liver due to cirrhosis.

Slowing progression of the disease

There's no cure for cirrhosis, and the damage to your liver often is irreversible. However, the disease typically develops gradually and there are a variety

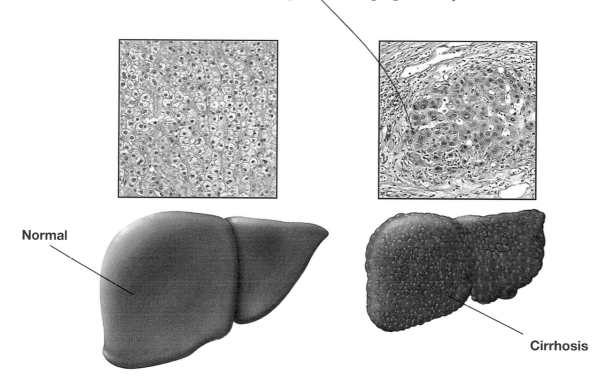

Normal

Cirrhosis

A normal liver (left), shown in cross section, shows no sign of scarring. The cirrhotic liver (right) shows extensive scarring and shrinkage.

of lifestyle changes you can make to reduce further damage.

Eat healthy and fresh

Cirrhosis tends to deplete your body of important nutrients. Fill your diet with plenty of fresh fruits and vegetables and whole-grain products that are high in fiber and nutrients, including vitamins C and E.

Your doctor also may prescribe supplemental vitamins K, A and D, because your body may not be getting adequate amounts. However, don't take any supplemental vitamins without your doctor's recommendation.

Restrict salt

The sodium in common table salt may cause you to retain fluid. So does cirrhosis. Reducing salt may be helpful in some people with liver disease to reduce fluid buildup.

Stop using alcohol

Alcohol breaks down into various chemicals when it's digested, and some of these substances are toxic to

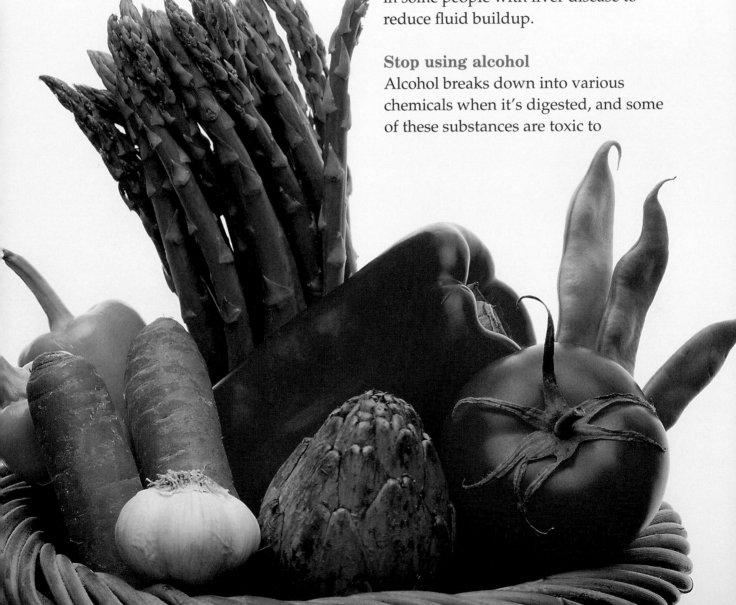

your liver. If you have cirrhosis, whatever the cause, avoiding alcohol will reduce the amount of waste your liver must process and help keep your liver healthier.

Limit medications

Your damaged liver cannot eliminate potentially toxic substances from medications in your system as it normally did. Discuss all medications you're taking, including nonprescription drugs, with your doctor. Be especially careful not to combine the pain reliever acetaminophen (Tylenol, others) or any other analgesic with alcohol, even if you take the drug only in the recommended daily amounts.

Avoid people who are sick

When your liver is damaged, you can no longer fight off infection as well as you did when your liver was healthy. Do everything that's reasonable to avoid getting sick. Start by getting vaccinated for hepatitis A and B, influenza and pneumococcal pneumonia.

Treating complications

Medical treatment for cirrhosis differs according to its cause and its signs and symptoms. In early-stage cirrhosis, it may be possible to minimize damage to the liver by treating the underlying cause, for example, alcohol dependency or hepatitis. For more advanced cirrhosis, the focus of medical care often is on treating complications of the disease.

Preventing internal bleeding

Cirrhosis can slow or block the movement of blood through your liver. This may cause the formation of small, twisted blood vessels (varices) with thin walls, most commonly in the esophagus or stomach. Because the walls are subject to high pressure, it's not uncommon for the blood vessels to start bleeding.

To stop internal bleeding, your doctor may recommend a medication to help lower the pressure within the varices. Another option is an endoscopic procedure using rubber band ligation to stop blood from flowing into the varices.

Reducing fluid retention

Diuretics may be used to help reduce the accumulation of excess fluid in your abdomen. Your doctor also may ask you to restrict sodium intake, including cutting down on table salt, to reduce fluid retention.

Sometimes, fluid that builds up in your abdomen can become infected, causing pain and fever. If this occurs, your doctor may insert a catheter into the abdomen to remove a fluid sample. Laboratory analysis of the sample can help identify the infecting organism and the proper antibiotic can be prescribed.

Reducing itching

Antihistamines as well as cholestyramine (Questran) may be prescribed to reduce itching caused by toxins (bile acids) in your blood.

Treating hepatic encephalopathy

In advanced cases of cirrhosis, you may become confused and delirious or go into a comatose state. This condition, called hepatic encephalopathy, occurs because your brain has come under assault from toxins in your blood, such as ammonia, that are normally eliminated from your body by a healthy liver.

Infection and bleeding into the gastrointestinal tract can cause episodes of hepatic encephalopathy. Treatment usually requires locating the source of infection or bleeding and treating it. In addition, you may be asked to take lactulose, either orally or as an enema. This medication can increase bowel movements and help remove ammonia and other toxins from your body.

Your doctor may also recommend an antibiotic to reduce certain bacteria in your intestines that produce ammonia. This will help lower the toxic levels of ammonia.

Chapter 14

Cancer

Cancer has the reputation of a virulent, incurable disease. The truth is that, although cancer remains a very serious illness, it's no longer the inevitable death sentence it once was. Being diagnosed with cancer is increasingly a tale of survivorship.

Worldwide, millions of people are alive today after having survived cancer. The cancer death rate is steadily declining, and the rate of new cancer cases is dropping. But the fight is far from over. Annually, cancer is diagnosed in approximately 1.5 million Americans, including estimates of over 140,000 cases of colon and rectum (colorectal) cancer and 43,000 cases of pancreatic cancer. In the United States, cancer causes more than 500,000 deaths each year — nearly 1 of every 4 deaths.

When digestive signs and symptoms occur, the first thing people often fear is cancer. Most of the time, cancer isn't the cause — but sometimes it is. Signs and symptoms such as bleeding, difficulty swallowing, unexplained weight loss and a change in bowel habits can be warning signs of cancer.

Why cancer develops in some people and not in others isn't fully understood, but researchers are learning about factors that may contribute to its onset. They know that most cancers develop slowly, and the symptoms often don't appear until the disease is established. Regular screening tests may be the best approach to detecting cancer at an early and most treatable stage. Generally, these test results only hint at rather than confirm that the cancer is present.

You may wonder, "Why even bother with screening tests if you can't be sure?" Typically, these tests are part of a general physical exam, and they tend to be simple, painless and inexpensive. What they provide is an early alert for something that you would otherwise be unaware of.

Why is that important? In most cases, the earlier a cancer is detected, the greater the chances are that it can be treated. Your doctor can design a treatment plan based on the nature of the cancer and the extent of its spread in your body.

What is cancer?

There are at least 200 different kinds of cancer, and most are associated with a specific organ or tissue. But the basic characteristic of all cancers is the same — the uncontrolled growth and spread of abnormal (malignant) body cells.

In your body, new cells are created to replace injured or dead ones through a controlled process of cell division called mitosis. Your body's function and good health depends, in part, on the balance between mitosis and the process of natural cell death called apoptosis.

Unlike healthy cells, cancer cells either lack the controls that switch off growth or lose their ability to undergo apoptosis. They divide without restraint, crowding out neighboring cells and competing for available nutrients, interfering with normal body functions.

A result of uncontrolled cell growth is often a densely packed mass of excess tissue called a tumor. These nodules can press on nerves, block arteries, bleed, obstruct the intestinal tract or interfere with the work of nearby organs.

Cancer cells can also travel to other parts of the body via the bloodstream or lymphatic system — a process called metastasis (muh-TAS-tuh-sis). When cancer spreads outside its place of origin, the disease becomes much more lethal and difficult to treat.

Not all cells that exhibit rapid or uncontrolled growth are cancer cells. Some cells may group together to form benign tumors, which typically don't damage the surrounding tissue, don't spread to other parts of the body and aren't life-threatening.

A complex mix of factors, including lifestyle, environment and heredity may be responsible for turning a healthy cell cancerous. Researchers theorize that most people have genes that can produce cancerous cells. These genes lie dormant until they're activated by an outside agent — such as an infection, sunlight, tobacco or pollutants in food, air or water.

You can get cancer almost anywhere, but most gastrointestinal cancers occur in the colon and rectum, where food waste moves slowly and toxins linger. The cancers most likely to occur in your digestive organs are:

Carcinomas

These cancers originate in the soft tissues that line your internal organs. Most cancers of the digestive tract fall into this category.

Lymphomas

These cancers develop in your immune system, especially the lymph nodes. You have clusters of lymph nodes in your neck, chest, underarms, abdomen and groin. Lymphatic tissue also exists in your intestines and within or near other internal organs.

Sarcomas

These cancers develop in connective tissues, such as muscle or bone. Smooth muscle, with its ability to stretch and contract, is common throughout the gastrointestinal tract.

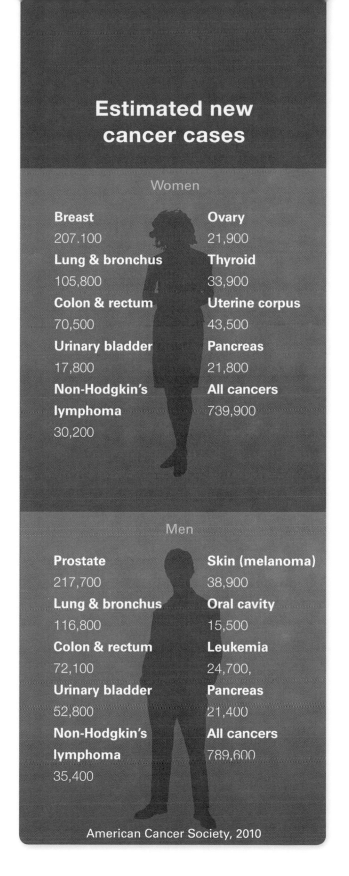

Estimated new cancer cases

Women

Breast	Ovary
207.100	21,900
Lung & bronchus	Thyroid
105,800	33,900
Colon & rectum	Uterine corpus
70,500	43,500
Urinary bladder	Pancreas
17,800	21,800
Non-Hodgkin's lymphoma	All cancers
30,200	739,900

Men

Prostate	Skin (melanoma)
217,700	38,900
Lung & bronchus	Oral cavity
116,800	15,500
Colon & rectum	Leukemia
72,100	24,700,
Urinary bladder	Pancreas
52,800	21,400
Non-Hodgkin's lymphoma	All cancers
35,400	789,600

American Cancer Society, 2010

Cancer of the esophagus

Cancer can develop anywhere in your esophagus. Researchers aren't certain of its cause, but your risk increases if you smoke or drink excessive amounts of alcohol. Barrett's esophagus, a complication of gastroesophageal reflux disease (GERD), is another risk factor (see pages 103-105). A diet low in fruits and vegetables also appears to increase risk. Men are nearly twice as likely to have esophageal cancer as are women.

Unfortunately, the small tumors that develop in your esophagus in early stages of the disease usually don't produce signs and symptoms. Often, the first indication of a tumor may be difficulty swallowing, when the tumor has grown to fill about half the opening of your esophagus. As the cancer develops, you may experience weight loss, chest pain and blood in vomit or stool. There are two types of esophageal cancer, based on the cells involved:

Squamous cell carcinoma
This cancer forms in flat, scaly (squamous) cells that line the entire length of your esophagus. Tobacco and excessive alcohol use increase your risk of this type of cancer.

Esophageal cancer
Key signs and symptoms

- Difficulty swallowing
- Blood in vomit or stool
- Weight loss
- Chest pain

Adenocarcinoma
This cancer develops in glandular tissue in your lower esophagus. People with severe acid reflux disease and Barrett's esophagus are at greater risk of this type of cancer.

Diagnosis

If you're experiencing signs and symptoms, the doctor may examine your esophagus for suspicious tissue or tumor growth with a barium X-ray. The doctor may also turn to endoscopy, in which a thin, flexible tube with an attached camera (endoscope) is inserted down your throat for closer inspection. The endoscope may collect a sample of tissue (biopsy) for lab inspection.

If cancer is identified, the next step is to determine how far the disease has spread. For this, your doctor may use blood tests and computerized tomography (CT) or endoscopic ultrasound. All of these tests are described in greater detail in Chapter 4.

There are no tests to screen for cancer of the esophagus, although periodic endoscopy and biopsies may be useful for people with Barrett's esophagus, which places them at increased risk.

Treatment

If your cancer is small and confined to the inner layers of the esophagus, your doctor may recommend removing the cancer with a margin of healthy tissue that surrounds it. This often can be done using an endoscope.

The most common treatment for esophageal cancer is removing the cancerous section and reconnecting the remaining healthy sections of your esophagus (esophagectomy). If a large portion must be removed, your surgeon may form a new passageway from throat to stomach using intestinal tissue.

Most often, surgery only reduces symptoms and may prolong survival. Eventually, the cancer recurs in most people. Your prognosis often depends on how much the cancer has spread.

Chemotherapy uses chemicals to kill cancer cells, while radiation therapy uses high-powered energy beams. Both therapies may be used, either alone or in combination, to ease symptoms, shrink the tumor or kill cancerous cells that have spread.

Other methods to destroy cancer cells include photodynamic therapy, which uses medications that make cancer cells sensitive to laser light, and radiofrequency ablation that uses high-energy waves to the same effect.

Stomach cancer

In the 1930s, stomach cancer was a leading cause of cancer death among American males. Since then, the incidence of stomach cancer has decreased dramatically, and improvements in food preservation may be why. Years ago, salting and smoking were common preservation methods, processes that could introduce cancer-causing substances to food. Today, most perishable foods are either frozen or refrigerated.

Improved socioeconomic status and sanitation practices also may have helped reduce the incidence of *Helicobacter pylori (H. pylori)* infection.

Stomach cancer
Key signs
and symptoms

- Upper abdominal pain
- Nausea and vomiting
- Loss of appetite
- Feeling full after eating only a moderate amount
- Blood in vomit or stool
- Weight loss

H. pylori is a bacterium associated with peptic ulcers and stomach cancer. Other factors that may increase your risk of stomach cancer include:

- Smoking
- Excessive alcohol use
- Family history of stomach cancer
- Small growths in the stomach lining (adenomatous polyps)
- Previous surgery to remove a portion of your stomach (partial gastrectomy)
- Vitamin B-12 deficiency (pernicious anemia) and associated wasting (atrophy) of the stomach lining

Most stomach cancers form in glandular tissues that line the stomach (adenocarcinomas). While stomach cancer is now much less common in the United States, in countries where smoking and salting are still widely used for food preservation and where *H. pylori* is more prevalent, stomach cancer remains a leading cause of cancer death.

Diagnosis and treatment

Barium X-ray and endoscopy are the most common tests for diagnosing stomach cancer. Endoscopic ultrasound and CT scanning may determine the spread of cancer into the stomach wall and adjacent tissues. For more on these procedures, see Chapter 4.

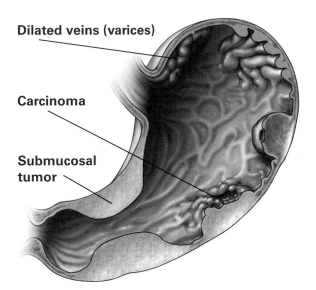

Dilated veins (varices)

Carcinoma

Submucosal tumor

In addition to carcinomas in soft tissue of the stomach lining, are dilated veins, or varices, which may cause bleeding. Swelling caused by a submucosal tumor in deep layers of the stomach wall narrows the opening.

When diagnosed and treated early, stomach cancer often can be cured. The three main treatments are surgery, chemotherapy and radiation therapy. Which treatment you receive depends on many factors, including the location and stage of the cancer and the state of your general health. Your prognosis for more advanced cancer will depend on the extent to which the cancer has spread from the tumor.

Surgery is the only way to cure some stomach cancers. The goal is to remove all of the cancerous tissue, along with a margin of the healthy tissue surrounding it. If your cancer has not spread, the surgeon may remove all or part of the stomach (gastrectomy) along with the lymph nodes.

If your cancer is more advanced, the surgeon may recommend removing a portion of the stomach primarily to relieve signs and symptoms, such as vomiting or bleeding.

Chemotherapy and radiation therapy can shrink tumors, making them easier to remove surgically. If the cancer is advanced, these therapies may relieve signs and symptoms and extend your survival. Some studies suggest they may also delay or prevent cancer recurrence following surgery.

Cancer of the small intestine
Key signs and symptoms

- Cramps
- Bloating
- Nausea and vomiting
- Blood in stool
- Weight loss

Cancer of the small intestine

Only a small percentage of all digestive cancers occur in the small intestine. The cause of this type of cancer is unknown, but you're at greater risk if you have Crohn's disease or a history of inflammation in the small intestine. Cancer of the small intestine is most often diagnosed in people between the ages of 50 and 60.

Diagnosis and treatment

Cancer of the small intestine typically has no signs and symptoms in its early stages. The cancer is most often detected in advanced stages after barium X-rays or a CT scan have been taken. Depending on the tumor's location, doctors may be able to remove a tissue sample (biopsy) using an endoscope.

Standard treatment for cancer of the small intestine is to surgically remove the cancerous tissue. If surgery isn't possible or it fails to stop the cancer from spreading, your doctor may recommend chemotherapy, radiation therapy or both to slow tumor growth and relieve your signs and symptoms. The prognosis for this type of cancer depends on how far cancerous cells have spread from the tumor.

Gallbladder and bile duct cancers

Gallbladder cancer is rare, but it's most likely to occur in women in their 60s or 70s with a history of gallstones. Your risk of gallbladder cancer is four to five times greater if you have gallstones. For unknown reasons, it seems the larger your gallstones are, the greater the risk.

Most gallbladder cancers are adenocarcinomas (in cells of the inner lining). When tumors are discovered early, your chance of finding a cure is good. But because the disease causes few signs and symptoms, it's rarely diagnosed in the early stages. When signs and symptoms do develop, they're generally a result of the cancer invading adjacent structures, such as the bile ducts, causing jaundice.

Cancer of the bile ducts (cholangiocarcinoma) may involve the network of tiny bile channels within the liver or occur in ducts located outside the liver. Primary sclerosing cholangitis, an inflammatory condition associated with ulcerative colitis, is a known risk factor.

Diagnosis and treatment

Early-stage cancer is often found incidentally during surgery to remove gallstones. Ultrasound imaging may identify gallbladder cancer, but often when the disease is in a late stage. Other imaging techniques, such as computerized tomography (CT), provide little help in detecting early-stage gallbladder cancer but may be useful in determining how advanced the cancer is.

Surgery to remove the gallbladder may cure early-stage cancer but is ineffective for the later stages. Once the cancer has spread beyond the gallbladder, treatment will focus on relieving pain and improving your quality of life through medications or radiation therapy.

Cancer of the bile ducts usually grows slowly, spreads gradually and is often not diagnosed until advanced stages. It's generally treated with surgery to remove the tumor. Treatment may also include chemotherapy or radiation therapy. If surgery isn't possible, your doctor may place a tiny tube (stent) to keep the cancerous duct open, preventing blockage and relieving jaundice.

The prognosis for gallbladder cancer and cancer of the bile ducts depends on how advanced the cancer is and the extent to which it has spread.

Liver cancer

In the United States, most cancer that occurs in the liver begins in another part of the body, such as the colon, lung or breast. Doctors call this metastatic cancer, rather than liver cancer. And this type of cancer is named after its place of origin — for example, metastatic colon cancer describes a cancer that began in the colon and has spread to the liver.

Primary liver cancer, the kind that originates in the liver, is one of the most common forms of cancer in the world but is uncommon in the United States. It often develops from hepatocytes, the most common cells in your liver.

Most people don't show signs and symptoms in early stages of the cancer. Primary liver cancer is two to three times as common in men as in women, and it typically occurs after age 50. These factors may increase risk:

- Cirrhosis
- Chronic hepatitis B infection
- Long-term exposure to aflatoxin, a toxin in contaminated food
- Exposure to the chemical vinyl chloride used to make plastics
- Long-term use of male hormones that increase muscle mass and strength (anabolic steroids)

Diagnosis

As with most other digestive cancers, primary liver cancer ordinarily produces few signs and symptoms in its early stage. By the time signs and symptoms do appear, the cancer is often beyond the chance for a cure, but not beyond treatment.

Blood tests to detect functional abnormalities and imaging tests — ultrasound, computerized tomography (CT) or magnetic resonance imaging (MRI) — are generally the first steps in diagnosing liver cancer. Taking a biopsy of liver tissue may not be necessary.

Treatment

The goal of any treatment for cancer is to remove the cancer completely — and surgery is often the most effective recourse. The decision will depend on the number, size and location of the tumors, and on how well your liver is functioning. If the tumors are small and have not spread beyond the liver, your doctor may be able to remove all of the cancerous tissue successfully.

For a limited group of people who meet specific health criteria, a liver transplant also may be an option. But that is also dependent on finding donated liver tissue, either from a deceased person or a live donor.

When surgery or transplant isn't possible, treatment may focus on preventing the tumor from growing or spreading further. In some cases, only comfort care is provided to relieve symptoms.

Treatments for liver cancer that may help relieve signs and symptoms and extend survival include:

- Blocking the main artery to the liver and injecting a chemotherapeutic drug in the sealed-off artery (chemoembolization)
- Injecting concentrated alcohol into the tumor to destroy cancer cells (ethanol ablation)
- Freezing the tumor with an instrument containing liquid nitrogen (cryosurgery)
- Heating the tumor with energy from high-frequency radio waves (radiofrequency ablation)

Traditional chemotherapy and radiation therapy may temporarily shrink liver tumors, but generally these procedures don't help people live longer. The prognosis for liver cancer depends on the extent that the tumor has spread.

Pancreatic cancer
Key signs and symptoms

- Abdominal and/or back pain
- Weight loss
- Yellowing of skin and eyes (jaundice)

Cancer of the pancreas

Although cancer of the pancreas accounts for only a small percentage of new cancer cases in the United States, it's the fourth-leading cause of cancer death — there were an estimated 36,800 deaths in 2010. The reason this cancer is so deadly is that it's usually diagnosed too late. Pancreatic cancer spreads rapidly outside the organ but is seldom detected in its early stages.

In addition, your pancreas is nestled among other organs deep in your abdomen, making it difficult for the doctor to detect a tumor by feeling (palpating) the area. Most pancreatic cancers develop in the lining of pancreatic ducts and grow undetected for a long time.

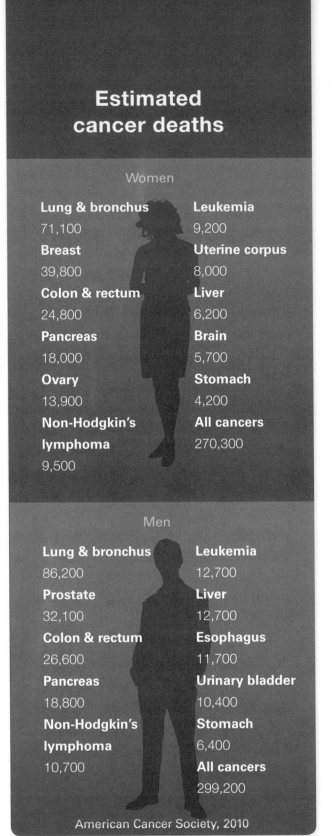

Estimated cancer deaths

Women

Lung & bronchus	**Leukemia**
71,100	9,200
Breast	**Uterine corpus**
39,800	8,000
Colon & rectum	**Liver**
24,800	6,200
Pancreas	**Brain**
18,000	5,700
Ovary	**Stomach**
13,900	4,200
Non-Hodgkin's lymphoma	**All cancers**
9,500	270,300

Men

Lung & bronchus	**Leukemia**
86,200	12,700
Prostate	**Liver**
32,100	12,700
Colon & rectum	**Esophagus**
26,600	11,700
Pancreas	**Urinary bladder**
18,800	10,400
Non-Hodgkin's lymphoma	**Stomach**
10,700	6,400
	All cancers
	299,200

American Cancer Society, 2010

Factors that may increase your risk of pancreatic cancer include:

- Smoking
- Age, especially if you're over age 60
- Being African-American
- Being obese
- Family history of pancreatic cancer
- Chronic inflammation of the pancreas (pancreatitis)
- Diabetes

Diagnosis and treatment

Imaging tests are the most common procedures for detecting pancreatic cancer, including ultrasound, computerized tomography (CT) and magnetic resonance imaging (MRI). If imaging reveals a tumor or provides some other evidence of cancer, the next step may be an ultrasound-guided endoscopy that removes a sample (biopsy) of pancreatic tissue for laboratory analysis.

If tests indicate that the cancer is confined to your pancreas, surgery to remove all or part of the organ may result in a cure. However, only a small number of surgeries completely remove all cancerous tissue. If cancer has spread outside the pancreas, surgery usually is not an option.

The Whipple procedure involves removing the head of your pancreas, parts of the small intestine and bile duct, and all of your gallbladder. Part of the stomach also may be removed. The surgeon reconnects the remaining parts of your pancreas, stomach and intestines to allow digestion to resume. Expect a recovery time of 10 days or more in the hospital and several more weeks at home.

Radiation therapy and chemotherapy don't cure the cancer but may help extend your survival. They can destroy cancer cells that remain following surgery and may help relieve pain and other symptoms. The prognosis for advanced pancreatic cancer depends on how far the cancer has spread.

Colorectal cancer

Colon cancer is cancer of the large intestine (colon) — the final portion of your intestinal tract — and rectal cancer involves the last several inches of the colon (rectum). Together, they're often referred to as colorectal cancer.

Colorectal cancer is the most common of all digestive cancers. In the United States, about 145,000 cases are diagnosed each year. Unlike many digestive cancers, the long-term survival rate is relatively good, provided the disease is caught early. The five-year survival rate for people treated in early stages is about 90 percent. Once the cancer spreads to adjacent lymph nodes, the survival rate declines sharply.

Most cases of colon cancer begin as noncancerous (benign) growths called polyps on the inside lining of the colon. The polyps may be small and produce few, if any, signs and symptoms. Over time, some polyps become cancerous. For more information on polyps, see page 235.

To help prevent colorectal cancer, doctors recommend regular screening tests that detect polyps before they become cancerous. However, many people don't take advantage of screening tests. That's one reason why colorectal cancer causes over 50,000 deaths in the United States each year, trailing only lung cancer as a leading cause of death from cancer.

Are you at risk?

As with other digestive cancers, heredity and lifestyle factors appear to play combined roles in the development of colorectal cancer.

Family history

You're at greater risk of colorectal cancer if a parent, sibling or child has the disease. The more family members that have it, the greater your risk. In some cases, this connection may not be due to hereditary but rather due to having a diet or lifestyle in common, for example, shared exposure to cancer-causing substances.

Research has identified several inherited conditions that are linked to colorectal cancer. Having one of these mutations wouldn't make cancer inevitable, but it would increase your individual risk significantly. The inherited conditions include hereditary non-polyposis colorectal cancer (HNPCC) syndrome, and familial adenomatous polyposis (FAP).

Colorectal polyps

Cellular changes can occur in the interior lining of the colon that often develop into noncancerous, or benign, growths known as polyps (adenomas, see page 233). Not all polyps will become cancerous, but almost all colon cancers start as polyps.

Previous colorectal cancer

Following treatment for colorectal cancer, polyps may develop at new locations that may become cancerous.

Race

African-Americans have a greater risk of colorectal cancer than do people of other races. They also tend to have it at a slightly earlier age.

Age

About 90 percent of people diagnosed with colorectal cancer are older than 50. The disease occurs in younger people but much less frequently.

Inflammatory intestinal conditions

A history of ulcerative colitis or Crohn's disease involving a substantial part of the colon increases your risk of colorectal cancer, and of developing it at a younger age.

Smoking

Research shows higher rates of colorectal cancer among people who smoke. The longer you smoke and the more tobacco you use, the greater your risk.

Diet

People with a high-fat diet, especially one containing a lot of red meat, have a higher risk of colorectal cancer. A diet high in fiber, on the other hand, has long been considered a way to lower your cancer risk. The role of fiber, however, is controversial, as recent studies suggest fiber may not protect against colorectal cancer at all.

Colorectal polyps — Early warning signs

The lining inside your colon is usually smooth. But some people have polyps, growths that sprout from the lining and intrude into the channel through which food waste passes. Many people will have one or more at any given time, but some people may have hundreds or thousands of polyps in their colons.

Your risk of having polyps increases with age — as many as 4 out of 10 people older than age 60 have them. Most polyps don't become cancerous, but some do.

The smaller the polyp, the less likely it is to be cancerous. The precancerous stage is a window of opportunity to detect and remove the growths, which your doctor can do relatively easily using an endoscope.

You should have a colonoscopy examination, or an alternative form of screening test, beginning at age 50. If you have a higher than average risk of colorectal cancer, your doctor may recommend that screening begin at an earlier age.

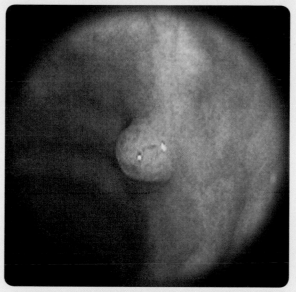

Polyps are small, noncancerous growths of various shapes and sizes that may develop in your colon and rectum.

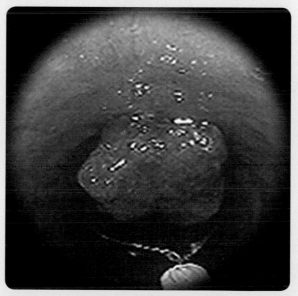

A polyp can be removed with a thin wire attached to an endoscope.

Inactivity

People who are inactive tend to be at increased risk of colorectal cancer. This may be related to obesity because people who are inactive also tend to be overweight.

Obesity

People who are obese are at increased risk of getting colorectal cancer and of dying of cancer when compared to people who are considered having a healthy weight.

Signs and symptoms

Many people with colorectal cancer experience no signs and symptoms in early stages of the disease. When they do appear, the signs and symptoms will likely vary depending on the origin of the cancer and the extent of its spread within your colon.

A cancer that's located in the lower portion of your colon or rectum can block the passage of stool, causing cramps. This also makes it difficult to have a bowel movement. You may frequently feel the urge to have a bowel movement and even after having one you may continue to experience an urge to have another. Blood in your stool or in the toilet bowl is another warning sign of colorectal cancer.

Cancer of the colon and rectum
Key signs and symptoms

- Blood in stool
- Change in bowel habits
- Abdominal pain
- Weight loss
- New-onset diabetes mellitus

Cancer in the upper portion of the colon can cause anemia, especially iron deficiency anemia, and fatigue due to blood loss that you may not be aware of or see. The blood may be masked because it's usually mixed in with stool and can be dark in color.

Other signs and symptoms of cancer in the upper portion of your colon include persistent diarrhea or constipation, decreased appetite, unexplained weight loss, and abdominal pain.

Be aware that any of these signs and symptoms may be caused by other medical conditions and not necessarily by colorectal cancer. Take any questions you have to the doctor and have any concerns checked and treated as early as possible.

Screening and diagnosis

The U.S. Preventive Services Task Force has strongly recommended that most people begin colorectal cancer screening at age 50. If you have other risk factors, such as a family history of colorectal cancer or polyps, or inflammatory bowel disease, you may benefit from earlier screening.

Screening tests allow your doctor to monitor the health of your colon and detect polyps or cancer in an early stage — before signs and symptoms appear. The tests, many of which are described in Chapter 4, include:

- Colonoscopy
- CT colonography
- Sigmoidoscopy
- Fecal occult blood test
- Colon X-ray (barium X-ray)
- Digital rectal exam

Colonoscopy is considered the gold standard for colon cancer detection. For this procedure, a thin, flexible tube with an attached camera is threaded through the colon, allowing your doctor to examine the interior lining of the colon for cancer or precancerous polyps. Removal of precancerous polyps will reduce your risk of colon cancer by more than 90 percent.

Staging cancer

If cancer is detected in the colon during screening tests, your doctor will decide what additional tests may be necessary. Unlike some other cancers, the size of the tumor is not a major factor in determining the outcome of colorectal cancer. Of greater importance is how far the cancer has spread. Called staging, this testing process determines your outlook and what treatment may be appropriate for your cancer.

The additional tests may include a physical exam, biopsies and a variety of imaging tests, such as computerized tomography (CT) or magnetic resonance imaging (MRI), which are described in Chapter 4. Surgery also may be a part of the staging process.

Primary factors that the doctor must take into account during the staging process are:

- To what extent has cancer spread through tissue layers of the colon wall, from the inner lining (mucosa) to the outer layer?
- Has cancer spread to nearby lymph nodes?
- Has cancer spread (metastasized) to organs in other parts of the body, such as the liver or lungs?

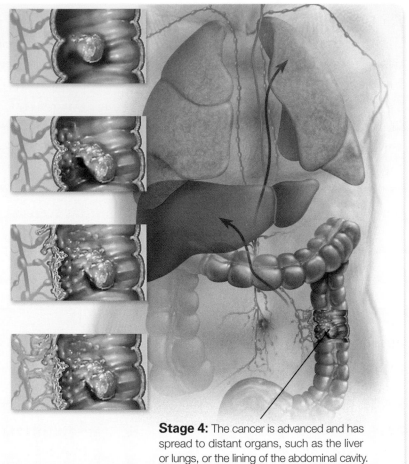

Stage 0: The cancer is in its earliest stage. It hasn't grown beyond the inner layer (mucosa) of the colon or rectum.

Stage 1: The cancer has grown through the mucosa but hasn't spread outside the colon wall.

Stage 2: The cancer has grown through the wall of the colon or rectum but hasn't spread to nearby lymph modes.

Stage 3: The cancer has spread to nearby lymph nodes but hasn't spread to other parts of the body.

Stage 4: The cancer is advanced and has spread to distant organs, such as the liver or lungs, or the lining of the abdominal cavity.

Unlike some other cancers, the size of the cancerous tumor isn't a major factor in determining the outcome of colorectal cancer. Of greater importance is how the cancer is spread.

When testing is complete, your doctor will categorize your cancer into one of five different stages. Each stage, from 0 to 4, indicates the spread of cancer on a scale of increasing severity:

Stage 0 indicates that the cancer is in an early stage and hasn't grown beyond the inner layer (mucosa) of the colon.

Stage 1 means the cancer has grown into the underlying tissue layers of the colon but hasn't spread outside the colon wall.

Stage 2 means the cancer has grown through the colon wall but has not spread to the lymph nodes. Your prognosis is still good at this stage.

Stage 3 means the cancer has grown through the colon wall and reached nearby lymph nodes but has not spread to other parts of the body.

Stage 4 means that the cancer has spread to an organ in another part of the body, such as the liver or lungs, or to the thin membrane lining the abdominal cavity.

Treatment

The type of treatment your doctor recommends will depend largely on what stage has been determined for your colorectal cancer. Your general health, other existing medical conditions, and the size and location of the tumor also may be factors.

Surgery, chemotherapy and radiation therapy are the primary treatments for colorectal cancer. You may have just one or all three forms of therapy.

For example, your treatment may differ slightly if the tumor is located in the colon or the rectum. Surgery, sometimes supported with chemotherapy, is the primary option for colon cancer. Surgery is also common for rectal cancer, sometimes supported with both radiation therapy and chemotherapy.

If the cancer is small, limited to a polyp, and in an early stage, your doctor may be able to remove the abnormal tissue during a colonoscopy (polypectomy). Larger polyps may be removed with laparoscopic surgery. Your surgeon performs the operation by inserting instruments through several small incisions rather than one large incision. The instruments are equipped with cameras to guide the procedure. Laparoscopic surgery generally has good results with a shorter hospital stay and, perhaps, less risk of complications.

If the cancer has grown into or through your colon, the surgeon may recommend a colectomy. This procedure removes the entire section of the colon containing the cancer, along with a margin of healthy tissue on each side. Nearby lymph nodes are usually also removed and tested for cancer.

Usually, the surgeon can reconnect the healthy portions of your colon or rectum. When that's not possible, a colostomy (kuh-LOS-tuh-me) may be necessary. This involves making an opening in the abdomen wall, providing a new path for waste to leave your body. The waste is collected in a special bag. A temporary colostomy is sometimes made to allow the colon or rectum to heal following surgery.

Radiation therapy or chemotherapy may be necessary to kill cancerous cells still present after surgery. For advanced cancer that can't be treated surgically, radiation therapy and chemotherapy are used to help shrink tumors, relieve symptoms and extend survival.

It's extremely important to schedule follow-up visits with your doctor after treatment. Small amounts of cancer cells sometimes can remain undetected in your body, allowing the disease to return. Regular checkups are useful for monitoring your health and detecting any changes that suggest a recurrence.

Additional resources

Contact these organizations for more information about digestive conditions. Some groups offer free material. Others have material you can purchase.

American Cancer Society
1599 Clifton Road NE
Atlanta, GA 30322
(800) 227-2345 or (404) 329-7942
www.cancer.org

American College of Gastroenterology
P.O. Box 342260
Bethesda, MD 20827
(301) 263-9000
www.acg.gi.org

American Dietetic Association
120 S. Riverside Plaza, Suite 2000
Chicago, IL 60606
(800) 877-1600 or (312) 899-0040
www.eatright.org

American Gastroenterological Association
4930 Del Ray Ave.
Bethesda, MD 20814
(301) 654-2055
www.gastro.org

American Hemochromatosis Society
4044 W. Lake Mary Blvd.
Unit 104, PMB 416
Lake Mary, FL 32746
(888) 655-4766 or (407) 829-4488
www.americanhs.org

American Institute for Cancer Research
1759 R St. NW
Washington, DC 20009
(800) 843-8114 or (202) 328-7744
www.aicr.org

American Liver Foundation
75 Maiden Lane, Suite 603
New York, NY 10038
(212) 668-1000
www.liverfoundation.org

American Pancreatic Association
P.O. Box 14906
Minneapolis, MN 55414
(612) 626-9797
www.american-pancreatic-association.org

American Society of Colon and Rectal Surgeons
85 W. Algonquin Rd., Suite 550
Arlington Heights, IL 60005
(847) 290-9184
www.fascrs.org

American Society of Gastrointestinal Endoscopy
1520 Kensington Rd., Suite 202
Oak Brook, IL 60523
(866) 353-2743 or (630) 573-0600
www.asge.org

Canadian Celiac Association
5025 Orbitor Drive
Building 1, Suite 400
Mississauga, ON L4W 4Y5
Canada
(905) 507-6208 or (800) 363-7296
(Canada only)
www.celiac.ca

Celiac Disease Foundation
13251 Ventura Blvd., Suite 1
Studio City, CA 91604
(818) 990-2354
www.celiac.org

Celiac Sprue Association
P.O. Box 31700
Omaha, NE 68131
(877) 272-4272 or (402) 558-0600
www.csaceliacs.org

Centers for Disease Control and Prevention
1600 Clifton Road
Atlanta, GA 30333
(800) 232-4636
www.cdc.gov

Children's Digestive Health and Nutrition Foundation
1501 Bethlehem Pike
P.O. Box 6
Flourtown, PA 19031
(215) 233-0808
www.cdhnf.org

Colon Cancer Alliance
1200 G St. NW, Suite 800
Washington, DC 20005
(877) 422-2030 or (202) 434-8980
www.ccalliance.org

Crohn's and Colitis Foundation of America
386 Park Ave. S
17th Floor
New York, NY 10016
(800) 932-2423
www.ccfa.org

Gluten Intolerance Group of North America
31214 124th Ave. S
Auburn, WA 98092
(253) 833-6655
www.gluten.net

The Hemochromatosis Information Center

2722 Wade Hampton Blvd., Suite A
Greenville, SC 29615
(864) 292-1175
www.hemochromatosis.org

Hepatitis Foundation International

504 Blick Drive
Silver Spring, MD 20904
(800) 891-0707 or (301) 622-4200
www.hepfi.org

Iron Disorders Institute

P.O. Box 675
Taylors, SC 29687
(888) 565-4766 or (864) 292-1175
www.irondisorders.org

Iron Overload Diseases Association

525 Mayflower Road
West Palm Beach, FL 33405
(561) 586-8246
www.ironoverload.org

International Foundation for Functional Gastrointestinal Disorders

P.O. Box 170864
Milwaukee, WI 53217
(888) 964-2001 or (414) 964-1799
www.iffgd.org

The Lustgarten Foundation

(for pancreatic cancer research)
1111 Stewart Ave.
Bethpage, NY 11714
(866) 789-1000 or (516) 803-2304
www.lustgarten.org

National Cancer Institute

Office of Communications and Education
6116 Executive Blvd.
Suite 300
Bethesda, MD 20892
(800) 422-6237
www.cancer.gov/cancerinfo

National Digestive Disease Information Clearinghouse

2 Information Way
Bethesda, MD 20892
(800) 891-5389
www.digestive.niddk.nih.gov

National Institute of Diabetes & Digestive & Kidney Diseases

Office of Communications and Public Liaison
NIDDK, NIH
Building 31, Room 9A06
31 Center Dr., MSC 2560
Bethesda, MD 20892
(301) 496-3583
www.niddk.nih.gov

The National Pancreas Foundation
101 Federal St., Suite 1900
Boston, MA 02110
(866) 726-2737
www.pancreasfoundation.org

**North American Society for Pediatric
Gastroenterology, Hepatology and Nutrition**
P.O. Box 6
Flourtown, PA 19031
(215) 233-0808
www.naspghan.org

Tri-County Celiac Support Group
TCCSG Shopping Guide
47819 Vistas Circle
Canton, MI 48188
www.tccsg.com

**United Ostomy Association
of America**
19772 MacArthur Blvd., Suite 200
Irvine, CA 92612
(800) 826-0826
www.uoa.org

Index

bacteria, 21–23
Crohn's disease, 143
defined, 21
descending, 21, 23
IBS disorder affecting, 130
illustrated, 15, 23, 143
sections, 21
sigmoid, 21, 23
transverse, 21, 23
ulcerative colitis, 143
X-ray, 80–81
See also colorectal
cancer
colonic transit, 94
colonoscopy
CT and, 87
defined, 86
in IBS diagnosis, 148
illustrated, 86
procedure, 86–88
as screening test, 88, 235
uses, 86
virtual, 87
See also diagnostic tests
colorectal cancer, 231–238
IBD and, 156
defined, 231
diagnosis, 235
polyps, 231, 233
polyps removal, 237
risk factors, 231–234
screening tests, 231, 235
signs and symptoms, 234
staging, 235–237
treatment, 237–238
tumor size and, 235, 236
colostomy, 178

complete blood count, 77
computerized tomography
abdominal, 82
in cirrhosis diagnosis, 217
colonoscopy, 87
defined, 81
and diverticulitis, 174
and gallstones, 187
illustrated, 80, 82
and pancreatitis, 196
procedure, 82
in staging colorectal
cancer, 235
constipation
causes, 67–68
defined, 67
as hemorrhoid cause, 71
medications for, 67
reasons to see doctor, 68
self-care, 68–69
corticosteroids
as hepatitis treatment,
208–209
as IBD treatment, 150
coughing, and GERD, 100
counseling, for IBS, 140
cox-2 inhibitors, 48
Crohn's disease, 141–158
B-12 shots, 153
bleeding, 70, 146
cause of, 144
colon cancer risk and, 156
colon illustration, 143
complications, 146
cramping and vomiting,
145
defined, 142

diagnosing, 148
diarrhea, 145
diet, 154–155
fistulas, 146
information and support,
156–157
medications for, 153
severity, 145
signs and symptoms,
145–146
stress reduction, 155
surgery for, 157
ulcers, 146
weight loss, 146
See inflammatory bowel
disease (IBD)
cryosurgery, 229
cyclosporine (Sandimmune),
151
cytoprotective agents, 124–
125

D _____

dairy products
limiting with IBD, 154
protein, 31
deep breathing, 136, 137
dermatitis herpetiformis, 162
diabetes
as GERD risk factor, 102
pancreatitis and, 193
treating, 199
diagnostic tests, 75–94
ambulatory acid (pH) probe
test, 90–91
blood tests, 76–77
capsule endoscopy, 88–89

risk factors, 224

signs and symptoms, 224

treatment, 225

stool

defined, 21

fluids as softener, 35

in rectum, 23

softeners, 138

stool antigen tests, 122

stool tests

DNA, 78

fecal occult blood test, 77–78

HemoQuant test, 78

purpose, 77

stress

constipation and, 69

diarrhea and, 66

digestive problems and, 25

effects on digestion, 46

IBS and, 131

nonulcer dyspepsia and, 127

peptic ulcers and, 125, 126

tolerance, 26

stress management, 46

for IBD, 155

for IBS, 136–137

strictures, 75

sulfasalazine (Azulfidine), 149

surgery

for colorectal cancer, 237

for diverticulitis, 177–178

as dysphagia treatment, 52

for gallbladder cancer, 227

for GERD, 112–114

for IBD, 157–158

for stomach cancer, 225

weight-loss, 43

swallowing difficulty, 51–53

T

tissue stretching for dysphagia, 52

tobacco. *See* smoking

transferrin saturation test, 213

transit studies

colonic transit, 94

defined, 92

gastric emptying, 92

gastric emptying and small bowel transit, 93

whole-gut transit, 93–94

tumor necrosis factor (TNF), 151

U

ulcerative colitis, 141–158

bleeding, 70

cause of, 144

colon cancer risk and, 156

colon illustration, 143

defined, 142

diagnosing, 148

diet management, 154–155

information and support, 156–157

nicotine gum and patches, 152

medications, 149-153

severity, 147

signs and symptoms, 147

stress reduction, 155

surgery for, 157–158

See inflammatory bowel disease (IBD)

ulcers

with Crohn's disease, 146

defined, 102, 116

duodenal, 116

esophageal, 103

gastric, 116

pressure, 116

signs and symptoms, 115

types of, 116

See also peptic ulcers

ultrasound

cirrhosis diagnosis, 217

defined, 83

endoscopic, 89–90

gallstone diagnosis, 186–187

illustrated, 83

pancreatitis treatment, 196

uses, 83–84

See also diagnostic tests

upper endoscopy, 84–85

defined, 84

illustrated, 85

for GERD diagnosis, 106

for peptic ulcer diagnosis, 120

upper gastrointestinal X-ray

defined, 79

for GERD diagnosis, 106

procedure, 79

See also X-ray

urine tests, 77

ursodiol (Actigall), 189–190

V

vegetables, 28–29, 30
virtual colonoscopy, 87
vomit
    blood in, 70
    with Crohn's disease, 145
    nausea and, 61–62

W

waist circumference, 39
water, drinking, 35, 60
        See also fluids
weight loss
    activity increase for, 43
    approach, 40–43
    calorie burn table, 42
    commitment, 40, 43
    with Crohn's disease, 146
    as digestive complaint, 73
    and GERD, 107–108
    goals, 41
    medications for, 43
    need determination, 39–40
    positive thinking, 41
    priorities, 41
    starving oneself and, 41
    surgery, 43
    See also healthy weight
wheezing, as GERD symptom,
    100
Whipple procedure, 231
whole-gut transit
    defined, 93
    illustrated, 93
    procedure, 93–94
    See also diagnostic tests
Wilson's disease, 214

X

X-rays
    colon (barium enema), 80
    defined, 78–79
    in IBD diagnosis, 148
    small intestine, 79–80
    upper gastrointestinal, 79
    See also diagnostic tests

Y

yogurt, lactose intolerance
    and, 59

Z

Zollinger-Ellison syndrome,
    102